The Flying Child

A Cautionary Fairy Tale for Adults

*Finding a purposeful life after
Child Sexual Abuse
through compassionate and creative therapy*

Sophie Olson
Patricia Walsh

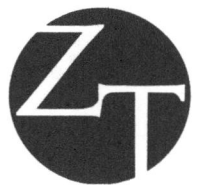

Praise for *The Flying Child*

This is a powerful and inspiring account of one person's journey to recovery after childhood abuse. It gives hope to us all.
– Dr Lucy Johnstone, Consultant Clinical Psychologist, Co-author of *The Power, Threat, Meaning Framework*

The mental health system declared Sophie disordered and irreparably ill, telling her that she'd never work again. This book - Sophie's story, serves as a vehement rejection of psychiatry's labels, and is a passionate testimony that true healing lies in relationship and connection.
– Jo Watson, author of *Drop the Disorder: Challenging the Culture of Psychiatric Diagnosis*

The Flying Child bravely depicts an unapologetically honest account of the devastating impact of child sexual abuse. It is a stark reminder of the need for us all to work towards creating a society where safe adults are appropriately equipped to act on concerns and give children the opportunity to speak out. It also highlights the significant need for those who have experienced abuse to have access to appropriate, trauma-informed support at the earliest opportunity. A powerful and courageous account, providing valuable insight for professionals.
– Kate Regan, NSPCC Team Manager

Sophie's book is an essential read for any adult working with children and young people, in schools, colleges, healthcare or the wider community. Sophie's story sensitively charts her own traumatic experiences and their long-term implications, reinforcing the absolute imperative that professionals should become informed about childhood sexual abuse. It reminds us to prioritise keeping children safe, prompts us to think the unthinkable, and shows us that any child could be suffering in silence. I hope this book helps to bring an end to childhood sexual abuse by highlighting its devastating consequences. It is our responsibility to notice children like Sophie, provide a safe space for them to be heard, and enable them to fly.
– Dr Clare Brunet, Headteacher

It's impossible to read Sophie Olson's account of her life after sexual abuse without being struck by her courage. But this book offers so, so much more - incredible skill and creativity, immense wisdom and psychological insight, inspiration, honesty, humility, and curiosity. A hunger not just for recovery, but for meaning. A desire to tell not just Sophie's story, but to leave every reader understanding themselves, their relationships and their world with greater depth, nuance, and – despite the pain of the subject – hope.

And there's love. Because this is also a story about the relationship between Sophie and her therapist, Patricia Walsh. It's a story of how professional compassion, commitment and courage can underpin healing; how integrity and creativity can elevate professional practice into a transformational experience for everyone involved.

In short – this is a very important book. Whether you're a survivor of trauma or a therapist, whether you seek or offer healing, whether you simply want to understand humans, our capacity for harm and for recovery; or whether you're an artist who wants to witness art in a living context at its raw and powerful best.

For Sophie and Patricia, creativity is activism, medicine, language, and life force. For these reasons, and for the love, the honesty, the beauty, and the hope - most of all the hope - I am grateful to them for the gift of this wonderful book.
– Clare Shaw, Writer, and Activist

The Flying Child – A Cautionary Fairy Tale for Adults *is a courageous, powerful, and thought-provoking book about healing after Child Sexual Abuse and the harms caused in the aftermath of abuse by systems unprepared to respond to trauma. It illustrates the importance of bearing witness to Child Sexual Abuse survivors' experiences, and the power of the wisdom held by survivors*
– Dr Síofra Peeren, Institute of Psychiatry, Psychology and Neuroscience, King's College London

The Flying Child *is a remarkable, compelling and urgent book. Sophie Olson has harnessed the fairy tale in the most ingenious and relatable way to portray the horror of her childhood, adolescence, and her journey into adulthood.*

Her writing is clear and clever, honest and evocative, and witnessing the abuse she suffered for so long broke my heart over and over.

Sophie's brilliance is to weave the threads of her therapy throughout, alternating the chapters of fairy tale and reality. This exchange allows space to breathe, not least for the reader, and is especially helpful in providing an independent voice so that we can understand what Sophie is going through at each stage. The insight, care and guidance of the therapist is invaluable; showing us how the mind works, what our memories mean, how we process trauma, and crucially how we can find a way out of the dark.

– **Joe Gibson, survivor and author of *Seventeen: A Coming of Age Story***

In my role as Therapeutic Team Manager for a service offering healing interventions to children who have experienced child sexual abuse I was keen to read this book on many levels; I was seeking an opportunity to fully understand the long term impact of a child's experience, I was keen to learn how to strengthen our team's approach and I wondered how the book might support some of children in their own process.

The book is written in such a way that I felt I was alongside the healing journey, as if in a therapeutic attunement with the author and there is a core message in the initial pages that validates what we as a team try to advocate in terms of Child Sexual Abuse in the author's choice to not provide a 'trigger warning'. For me this removes the shame and secrecy that allows harm to remain undiscovered.

It was the use of metaphor in the book that I feel will have the most profound impact on my practice - in our work with children, some as young as 3, the therapists try to find creative methods to give them a voice; a way to explore their muddles and worries. The concept of fairytale enables the child's story to be told through characters that represent their subconscious thoughts and feelings and make sense of them at their own pace.

– **Clare Sullivan, Barnados**

The Flying Child *simultaneously locates the reader in humanity's darkest and brightest, most hopeful hour. Through recorded interactions between Sophie Olson and her therapist Patricia Walsh, we learn of the deep and awful trauma of sexual abuse in childhood. It is closer up than most readers will have ever experienced such abuse. It is uncomfortable and awful, nightmarish, and yet, we read on. We are aware that Sophie is doing the hardest work of all, travelling back and facing her abuser and so, reading on, strangely, feels like a supportive act. We are with Sophie, every step of the way. And on every step of the journey we are unendingly grateful for the presence of Patricia. Ultimately, despite the book's difficult subject matter, we are buoyed by the strength of these two remarkable women: Sophie in persisting through a living hell; and Patricia in guiding her steadfastly back to her own strength and inner beauty. I have learned so much about the devastating impact of trauma from this book but I have learned more about the beauty, and the twinned fragility and strength of survivors.*

– Jenny Horgan, author, Columnist Irish Examiner, teacher

Although there are many memoirs that recount childhood abuse, some rely on familiar tropes. But this wonderful collaboration between Sophie Olson and Patricia Walsh is quite different. It is emotional but not sentimental, engaging as well as elevating. Through its different modes of telling – personal reflections, texts between survivor and therapist, the fairy story, the illustrations – it draws the reader to 'travel alongside' Olson. A precious resource for practitioners who want to deliver better services and for survivors and their allies alike.

– Dr Ruth Beecher, social and cultural historian, Birkbeck, University of London

Have you ever read a book and felt that it was an absolute privilege? That is how I feel after reading A Cautionary Fairy Tale for Adults. *A contained and delicate relational dance that enabled the deconstruction of shame and reclamation of power and hope. Sharing their journey, Sophie and Pat have allowed insight into the most private therapeutic process, demonstrating the power of words, courage and offer*

of a human interaction. It has a universal application for personal or professional development. Whatever your reason is for turning these pages, it will reach you in ways that you are not expecting, it provides a prism of perspective of the complexities of child abuse and the legacy of trauma that it leaves. Expect incitement, clarity, guidance, reflection, ideas and empowerment. The current safeguarding and trauma healing system must recognise that a child is not responsible for stopping their abuse and people must be reached at where they are at. If you are a curious and determined relational human and want to be part of the solution of human suffering, then start by reading this book. "The only option is to dare."
– Sarah Pritchard, Consultant Social Worker and Trainer

This book is an honest account of healing from childhood sexual abuse. Sophie breaks the silence that often surrounds this topic to share her experiences in a creative way. Her openness and honesty give the reader a deep insight into the challenges she faced on the road to healing. Whereas Pat offers the reader an understanding of the role a therapist can play in such a journey. This book gives readers a rare opportunity to see some of the ups and downs of a client-therapist relationship. Sophie's road to healing is a complex one, but this story is one of survival, healing, and activism. The use of creative story telling through fairy tales, metaphor and imagery shows an alternative way to conceptualise trauma that doesn't pathologize the survivor and instead focuses on hope and a journey of healing. This is a book about overcoming shame, and ultimately a story about the power of relationships.
– Dr Peter Blundell Senior Lecturer in Counselling and Psychotherapy Practice Liverpool John Moores University, UK, social worker, and psychotherapist

First published in the UK in 2024 by ZunTold
www.zuntold.com

Text copyright © Sophie Olson and Patricia Walsh 2024
Cover illustration:
"Nachtflug" in: Quint Buchholz,
Sonne, Mond und Abendstern
©1997 Carl Hanser Verlag
GmbH & Co.KG, München
Arranged for book cover purposes by Isla Bousfield-Donohoe

The moral right of the author has been asserted.
All rights reserved.
Unauthorised duplication contravenes existing laws.

A catalogue record for this book is available
from the British Library

ISBN 978-1-9157580-5-7
1 2 3 4 5 6 7 8 9 10

Printed and bound by Interak, Poland

Contents

A Cautionary Note	3
Foreword	5
Introduction	11
In the Beginning	15
PART ONE: Behind the Door	17
Catalyst	19
Coffee Mornings	26
A Small Taste of Activism	30
Two Steps Forward, One Step Back	32
Safeguarding	36
Therapy with Pat Begins	39
Behind the Big Black Door	46
Try Writing It as a Fairy Tale	51
The Kingdom of His	53
Exploring 'The Kingdom of His'	56
The Old Witch	58
Exploring 'The Old Witch'	60
The Butterfly Queen	63
Exploring 'The Butterfly Queen'	66
PART TWO: Acknowledgement	69
Standing on the Precipice	71
Flashbacks	78
All the Wrong Things	79
Planning	83
Exploring 'Planning'	85
Mind Capture	86
Exploring 'Mind Capture'	88
The Escalator and the Red Boots	91
Exploring 'The Escalator'	94
The Cage	97
Exploring 'The Cage'	101
We Are Not Nervous Patients	102

PART THREE: Believing, and the Struggles It Brings	107
Entering the Innermost Cave	109
Mind Capture (Part 2)	114
I Don't See Much Point to This Anymore	115
There Is Something Wrong With Me	123
Fighting the Demon	127
You Are Never Back Where You Started	130
Turning Out the Lights	132
No-God Who Art In Heaven	134
Exploring 'No-God Who Art In Heaven'	136
Dream Telling	142
Moving Mountains	148
Rules	150
Rules (Part 2)	153
Exploring 'Rules'	156
The Common	159
Exploring 'The Common'	162
Fragments	165
Opening the Big Black Door	170
The Lay-By	172
Exploring 'The Lay-by'	175
Blood and No Tears	176
The Touch	178
Exploring 'The Touch'	180
Am I Attracting Darkness?	181
Exploring	186
Exploring 'Exploring'	188
Exploring (Part 2)	189
Exploring 'Exploring (Part 2)'	191
Exploring (Part 3)	193
Gathering	195
Summertime	197
Exploring 'Summertime'	200
A Little While After	204
Exploring 'A Little While After'	206
Campervan and Saxophone	207
Processing and Writing	212
The Best You Can Do	214
Do You Think I am Strong Enough?	217
Dreams	219
Re-writing 'Summertime'	222

Telling My Story As 'I'	225
Detachment	229
Remembering the Basement	234
The Basement	237
Exploring 'The Basement'	240
Processing 'The Basement'	245
PART FOUR: Integration	**251**
Becoming Whole	253
School	258
Exploring 'School'	260
You're So Lucky	263
Exploring 'You're So Lucky'	266
The Shadow of Rocks	267
Exploring 'The Shadow of Rocks'	269
Is He Really a Monster?	270
Fourteen	271
Exploring 'Fourteen'	278
The Phone Call	282
Exploring 'The Phone Call'	286
Working with Anger and Grief	288
Repercussions: Sleeping Sickness	292
When the Darkness Descends	294
Adulthood	295
The Person In Charge	296
Repercussions: Grey	299
Triggering Event	302
Turning Dark	308
Exploring 'Turning Dark'	310
Beautiful Boy	315
Exploring 'Beautiful Boy'	319
PART FIVE: Rebuilding	**321**
The Mission and the Purpose	323
Manuscript Replies	325
Talk About The Flying Child Project	329
The Power of Art	330
Time to Create Change	336
The Flying Child	338

PART SIX: Consolidation	341
What the Doctors Didn't See	343
Severe and Enduring	350
Exploring 'Severe and Enduring'	353
Intergenerational Trauma	356
Bearing Witness	357
The Angry	359
Exploring 'The Angry'	361
The Journey	365
The White Witch and the Blossom Tree	369
The Women and the Purpose	373
Epilogue	381
Acknowledgements	387

This book is dedicated to the 'The Women' for teaching me we were not broken after all, and the millions of survivors of child sexual abuse across The World, many of whom I'm proud to call my friends. May your words turn into pink blossom trees, the people of The World watch and wonder, and may this world become a safer place for the children who live in it.

In memory of those no longer here, because of Child Sexual Abuse.

A Cautionary Note

~

Silence is a defining trait of Child Sexual Abuse. I decided against using the term 'trigger warning' because it would suggest my words are a loaded weapon, the implication being they are too dangerous to be spoken at all. A term designed to protect, it conditions us into believing stories like mine are too shameful or potentially damaging to others to risk speaking aloud.

My words are an important and valid expression of the harm done to me by others. They are not the danger. People who choose to sexually abuse children are the danger. They are the ones who should come with trigger warnings but of course we don't know who they are. They walk among us. They hide in plain sight, comfortable with the societal silence. Stories like mine that shatter silence send an important message – survivors can and will speak freely.

I acknowledge that some survivors find trigger warnings useful, and so will say this book contains references to Child Sexual Abuse and emotional abuse.

Because it is important for professionals to make the link between CSA and the often-devastating impact on mind, body, and soul, it also gives a raw and honest account of the times in my life I reached rock bottom. There are references to addiction, disordered eating, self-harm, and suicide.

The intention is not to demoralise or be gratuitous, it is for my story to make sense.

Many survivors seek support when they reach this point. Some, like me, will find it impossible to find the words to explain *why*. The professional or practitioner, without much needed context, is then left with both visible 'symptoms' to treat rather than an understanding of the root cause. This book brings context.

A Cautionary Note

Many of the references to CSA are metaphorical, but not all. The most graphic descriptions of abuse are removed because I know stories like mine can appeal to perpetrators of abuse and I will not allow my story to be used as fodder, so if that is why you are reading the book, you won't find what you're looking for here. You will, however, see that much work is being done to make the world a safer place for children, and you can no longer safely rely on silence.

Please take care when reading and take steps to look after yourself and remember this book is not intended to be used as a manual. How Pat worked was unique to me. She will work with other clients in ways unique to them and that's the point. Survivors are all different. Our abuse is different, how we survive is different and our needs will be different. Take it slowly, take a break or step away if you need to, have a cup of tea, wrap yourself in a comforting blanket, cuddle your dog, check in with yourself along the way.

Sophie Olson

Foreword
by Viv Gordon

~

Child Sexual Abuse (CSA) is a global epidemic. In the UK, there are an estimated 11 million adult CSA survivors[1] and 15% of girls and 5% of boys are growing up experiencing sexual abuse[2]. We are a huge, hidden community, overrepresented in all of society's most excluded populations including those experiencing homelessness, addiction, disability, long term mental health needs and chronic health conditions. CSA survivors are caught between catastrophically broken systems that perpetuate abuse, fail to protect children and fail to deliver healing or justice. Mental health systems label, medicate, incarcerate, 'treat' and silence us. Retraumatising, victim-blaming criminal justice systems have effectively decriminalised child sexual abuse through inefficacy.

Campaigns such as A Disorder for Everyone[3] have rallied for many years against the culture of psychiatric diagnosis that pathologise normal human distress and normal responses to trauma, discrimination and inequality. The medical model individualises a systemic issue. It makes survivors the problem – we are 'ill', 'mad' and 'disordered'. We have to 'recover', be better, be more mindful and resilient. We are made wrong – not abuse, not perpetrators, certainly not a society that looks the other way while CSA happens on such an unbelievable scale.

Simultaneously, prosecution rates are disastrously low[4]. Survivors navigate invasive scrutiny and endless waits and adjournments.

---

[1] Child Abuse and Neglect in the UK, NSPCC, 2011, Radford et al
[2] Scale and Nature of Child Sexual Abuse Report, CSA Centre, 2021, Karsna and Kelly
[3] https://www.adisorder4everyone.com/
[4] The percentage of reported cases resulting in a conviction are 1% adult cases and 3% childrens cases – Scale and Nature of Child Sexual Abuse Report, CSA Centre, 2021, Karsna and Kelly

Where 'justice is served' we face insulting sentencing and compensation payments. In 2019, dental student Christopher Daniel walked free from Dumbarton Sheriff Court after being found guilty of sexually abusing a 6 year old girl over a two year period. He was not placed on the sex offenders register and has no criminal record. Sheriff Gerard Sinclair stated that a recorded conviction would have 'serious consequences in terms of the accused's future career'[5]. Note there is no mention of how this will impact the girl's future.

So many of us live through many years of confusion, suicidality, self injury, distressed eating, homelessness or addiction. Tragically, Sophie's account is far from unique – there are 11 million of these journeys unfolding across the UK as you read this and 500,000 are added every year[6]. If yours is one of them – I hope this book helps you know you are not alone. I hope you know your survival is heroic.

What does justice even look like in this context? My own activism centres social justice. CSA survivors experience hermeneutical injustice[7]. Stigma and cultural silence mean that historically we have not had the language and frameworks through which we can articulate and understand our experiences. Not being able to talk about CSA prevents survivors from taking collective action. When we break the silence, we contribute to a new lexicon which – one voice at a time – builds our community infrastructure for social change.

For this reason, Sophie's generous sharing of her story is of great value. Textbooks can tell us the abuse was not our fault but nothing role models innocence like a survivor standing up to be counted. The book celebrates the power of creativity to enable these explorations in all their complexity, specificity and nuance. Writing that which she was unable to say in the tenor of the fairy tale, with the distance of the third person narrative, enabled Sophie to reach into her past and build a new future. The approach will be familiar for anyone versed in creative,

---

[5] https://www.theguardian.com/uk-news/2019/jan/31/family-attacks-failure-to-punish-student-who-sexually-assaulted-girl

[6] Scale and Nature of Child Sexual Abuse Report, CSA Centre, 2021, Karsna and Kelly

[7] Epistemic Injustice: Power and the Ethics of Knowing, OUP, 2007, Miranda Fricker

therapeutic inner child work[8]. Sophie is able to retrieve the parts of herself that had been locked behind the 'Big Black Door'. All survivors have their own version of this door.

Culturally we have had no choice but to shut parts of ourselves away. Taboo forces us to compartmentalise to survive. We have internalised the stigma, bought into the shaming deficit model of the dominant cultural and medical paradigms leaving us unable to resist our continued oppression. There are alternatives. For the last decade, I have worked within a social model of disability – exploring for myself first and then alongside many others what access and inclusion looks like for us as CSA survivors, initiating a now shared drive for CSA survival to become a protected characteristic in recognition of the common marginalisations, discriminations and microaggressions we face as a community. We want and deserve statutory access across all sectors and legal frameworks within which we can challenge and transform inaccessible systems.

This book asks what effective psychological and emotional support could be for CSA survivors, tracing in stark detail the failures in mainstream mental health approaches in contrast to the life saving properties of peer support and Sophie and Pat's unconventional therapeutic relationship. The book is not a manual – for survivors or professionals – and should not be read as one. It is one woman's journey accompanied by one professional. Both have taken great personal and professional risks in the context of horribly imperfect systems. What worked here would not work for everyone. The approach would not be deliverable, sustainable or preferred in all contexts. The need is huge, the support sector under-resourced and many professionals are already at risk of burnout. Additionally many survivors, myself included, often find the clarity and predictability of conventional therapeutic boundaries deeply healing after all boundaries have been shattered in abuse.

For Sophie and Pat, the approach paid off and they continue their journey to become co-authors with a shared vision of a retreat centre in recognition that healing does not just happen in office hours. They are not alone in this. In 2022, Rape Crisis

---

[8] A key CSA-focussed text in this field is *Rescuing The Inner Child*, Souvenir Press, 1994, Penny Parks

England and Wales launched a 24/7 helpline for round the clock support for anyone aged 16+ who has experienced sexual violence at any point in their lives[9]. At the same time, many activists are working to develop communities of belonging and networks of allies – excellent but overstretched sexual violence services increasingly embrace groupwork alongside a groundswell in CSA survivor-led trainings, peer support, creative initiatives and spaces.

This book does pay great testament to the power of trust relationships. Abuse is a relational crime and healing is also, necessarily, relational. Like all relationships, Pat and Sophie's is unique and the views shared in the book must be contextualised in that way. They are not facts or universal truths. Be discerning as you read this book – take what resonates for you and disregard what doesn't, follow your instincts, when we disagree it helps us articulate our own thoughts and beliefs. The most important trust relationship we need to build, as survivors or indeed as therapists, is with ourselves. I am confident that in this book, you will find ideas, images, words and wisdom that will cradle you – revisit them, read them out loud so they can fill the air you breathe and hold them tight – they are breadcrumbs on pathways that lead us back to ourselves and closer to each other.

Viv Gordon is a Child Sex Abuse Survivor Artist Activist and Artistic Director of Viv Gordon Company CIC and arts and social justice organisation creatively campaigning for voice, visibility, community and leadership by, for and with CSA survivors aged 14+. www.vivgordoncompany.com

---

[9] A key CSA-focussed text in this field is *Rescuing The Inner Child*, Souvenir Press, 1994, Penny Parks

'The Dreamer awakes,
The shadow goes by
The tale I have told you,
That tale is a lie.
But listen to me,
Bright maiden, proud youth
The tale is a lie;
What it tells is the truth.'

Traditional folktale ending

Introduction

My name is Sophie Olson, and I am a survivor of Child Sexual Abuse. It's a sentence I never thought I would say out loud. What happened after my own abuse was in some ways as traumatising, if not more so, than the abuse itself. Being a silent adult survivor in a world that doesn't talk about Child Sexual Abuse is isolating. For many years I felt like I was the only one and totally alone. Carrying a burden as heavy as CSA with no idea of how to release the words pooled in my heart was a relentless effort.

How do survivors begin?

I certainly didn't know how to speak those words. It would mean revealing the 'real' me. Which secrets would I tell first? I had so many. The darkest secret of all was locked deep inside me, imprisoned along with my words, battened down with fear and barricaded with shame. I couldn't tell. I needed help, but how to talk about it without judgement? How to explain about my coping mechanisms, how they initially whispered promises of sweet relief but now pushed me to the brink? How to talk about the secret scars on my body? The stockpiling of pills? The numerous times I woke up the morning after, wondering why I could not die, wondering why me? How to tell of my long and involved plans to exit this world in the way that caused least grief and anguish to those I love? *Where to start?*

Speaking my secrets was unthinkable. Impossible. People would think I had lost my mind, which, in a way, I had. It was trapped in the past world of childhood.

I had survived and continued to survive by going far from myself, shutting down, cutting out, dissociating, whatever you want to call it. I pushed memories of abuse to the back of my mind where they sat like a malevolent, ticking bomb.

Abuse might not have broken me but silence and secrets – pretending – did.

In 2009, the bomb exploded. I had a breakdown and was admitted to hospital for four months. This madness of mine became official. In the mental health system, my distress, the trauma, fear and grief were pathologised. Negotiating my way through a system that had little understanding of trauma and the role it played in my breakdown, was one of the hardest things to do. I thought I'd be there forever. It was to be ten years before I turned my back on the mental health system.

Tell us why you do these things? the staff on the wards asked, but I wasn't safe enough to tell. The hospital wasn't safe. The patients certainly weren't safe. I stayed silent and kept my secrets to myself.

I am not mad, I would say to myself and to the nurses handing out medication. *I shouldn't be here.*

It's not up to us. Talk to your consultant next week, they would reply. *Just take the pills, dear.*

They're not working, I'd say, and over the weeks my consultant continued to ply me with medication for *the chemical imbalance in the brain.* A pill for each secret, a pill for every memory. Sedation for distress and chemical restraint for fear. I was told I was there voluntarily, but they *strongly recommended* I didn't leave as they would then *have to review that.*

You are unwell, they said. *You must take the pills.*

After a while my psychiatrist gave up on me and said I would never recover.

'*You have a severe and enduring mental illness. You will never recover or live without medication and community support.*'

He could have told me that it's *normal* for a cup to shatter when it's smashed on the floor. He failed to say there are different ways to mend; that with gentle hands, patience and love, cups can be glued back together again, and whilst they may not be exactly as they were, they will still be a cup.

I found these gentle hands in peer support. Connecting with other survivors enabled me to put some of my smashed pieces back together. Shared experience helped. Validation and a safe, contained space. Ginger and lemon tea and a Bourbon biscuit every Tuesday morning on the top floor of the Samaritans did more for me than a bucket load of pills ever had.

It was a group facilitated by Patricia Walsh and later she

became my therapist. Her hands were gentle too. She used them to guide me on a journey and she sat with me in darkness and searched for my missing bits – the puzzle of me – helping me glue them back together. She didn't leave my side. She was patient and wise, telling me over and over again how *normal* I was.

I would be more concerned if you weren't reacting like this, she said. *Look at what happened to you.*

Not once did she say I was sick, disordered or beyond help, instead she helped me dispel the secrets and expose the rotting, festering wound of abuse, and we cleaned it together and let it dry, scab and heal. She told me how my challenges could become my strengths and slowly, slowly, I was put back together until I was a functioning person again, albeit with extra cracks and lots of glue – but whole.

I knew that to survive I needed to say the words about what happened to me. Pat helped me find a way to express trauma and she helped me to release my soul, trapped under layers of shame and fear. *The Flying Child* was the name I gave to the external manifestation of this story I couldn't express in words. It is written as a fairy tale, on Pat's suggestion, simply because I couldn't express it as 'me'. Each chapter became an important part of the therapeutic process, and the chapters are interwoven throughout this book. The timeline of my story was pieced together towards the end of this writing process, with 'In The Beginning' being one of the final chapters I wrote for Pat. This was the only chapter based on family anecdote rather than memory and it is my interpretation of the story of my birth and near-death experience that I have been told many times.

Alongside the chapters, kept in their original, unedited form, are records of the communication between me and Pat. I made the decision not to include all the fairy tale chapters. Others, I am yet to write.

Pat and I worked together in face-to-face therapy sessions but also in between sessions by email, WhatsApp and phone calls. We have documented the therapeutic journey and included the writing and drawings I created to help me make sense of my experiences and to reconnect with myself. My therapy with Pat led me from fighting to die, to healing and living, from darkness to light. Most importantly it has led me to survivor activism and the setting up of my own non-profit organisation to challenge Child Sexual Abuse through peer support and professional training. This book shares an honest journey of healing from trauma, and from the 'mental illness' that was never an illness at all.

Prologue

In the Beginning

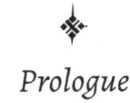

'Turn back, turn back, thou pretty bride,
Within this house thou must not abide.
For here do evil things betide.'

— *The Robber Bridegroom*, The Brothers Grimm

The Little Princess decided it was time to be born. It was far too early, but she had important work to do. One morning, at the very end of March, she knew she couldn't wait a moment longer and that her time had come.

Her body was new and so very small, but her soul was old and wise. She knew her Purpose was important, and she didn't know why or what it was, but she was keen to start. In her eagerness, she forgot to learn the basics.

One evening, whilst her mother, the Butterfly Queen, was giving her a bath, a drop of water fell into her mouth, and The Little Princess realised she hadn't yet learnt to cough because she was so small. The drop of water was huge in her tiny lungs, and it sat there. The Little Princess waited for it to continue its journey, but it didn't. It sat stubbornly and the Little Princess couldn't breathe.

I can't breathe, she thought to herself calmly and wondered where her next life would be. She watched with curious detachment as her mother, the Butterfly Queen fluttered and flew and pulled her tiny little body from the water. She watched her own little face turn blue and saw her mother, the Butterfly Queen, slapping her on the back.

Careful, she thought, followed by, *I still can't breathe.*

She watched the Butterfly Queen carry her little baby body

downstairs to a table, where a black telephone sat, and she watched with interest as the Butterfly Queen screamed and cried into the phone. She saw her big sister, the Big Princess, follow with a blanket, 'to keep the baby warm'. She felt with relief, the rush of air as the Butterfly Queen breathed for her, her mouth clamped over the Little Princess's tiny face, and then, there she was, back in her body once more.

She didn't like what happened after that.

She didn't like the prodding and the poking. The needles were sharp, and they hurt her, and she cried.

I don't like this, she tried to say as the biggest needle punctured her skin and stole the fluid that surrounded her spine, but she hadn't learnt how to speak, so no one understood.

I don't like this, she said, as she was put naked under big noisy machines, trying to find the answers she already knew.

I don't like this, she cried, as male hands held her when all she wanted was to be held by the Butterfly Queen, but no one listened, and no one understood her mewling. She started to worry that grown-ups were stupid.

The Little Princess understood that life would not be easy, and she felt a little worried. She didn't find it as easy to breathe as she had before, not because of a drop of water but because worry was getting in the way.

I survived though, she said, and waited for life to begin.

~ Part One ~

Behind the Door

Catalyst

Winter

When I contacted my local rape and sexual abuse charity for advice in 2016, I wasn't looking for peer support or therapy. I was looking for justice. I was resigned, after years of psychiatric treatment, never to 'recover' from Child Sexual Abuse.

Life wasn't *all* bad; I had moments of great joy and they came from motherhood. I loved being a mother but I was deeply unhappy, trapped in the revolving door of mental health services. My first inpatient stay was in 2009, followed by involvement from the community mental health team (CMHT), an extraordinary amount of medication, and ever-changing diagnostic labels from chronic depression to bipolar disorder.

The catalyst to seeking advice was the death of someone I knew. Her name was Frances Andrade. She had been comprehensively failed by the justice system. Our children had been in the same school, and when I finally came out of hospital, I remember bumping into her on the street and being surprised by her warmth. Despite the fact we didn't know each other well, she put her arms around me and gave me a big hug.

'I understand,' she said.

A few years later she died by suicide, after giving evidence in court, about non-recent sexual abuse by her former choirmaster. This news devastated me. I was aware of the trial as it was all over the media but had no idea I knew the victim. I saw her husband and child at the school gate and witnessed in their faces, the devastation suicide brings. I tried to explain to my own son why his friend's mother had died but I couldn't. Words failed me. I could not comprehend how it was that two women could make small talk for years about the weather, homework and other such insignificant things and not speak about the same burden we carried. How was this possible? How and why did we hide our trauma? I had the appalling sense of missed opportunity. I felt she had recognised something in me when we met that day. Would things have been different if either of us had said we were survivors of CSA? Possibly not, but the thought that we hadn't said anything, because we can't, because society tells us this subject is too unpalatable and because of our own underlying shame, was just too much to bear.

I knew then that, like her, I would also die and that my children would lose their mother too. This is why I picked up the phone and rang the helpline, because I was hit with the sudden and overwhelming need to *do* something about it. Therapy was the last thing on my mind. I could not face feeling misunderstood again.

I met with an ISVA (independent sexual violence advisor), as I wanted to report the abuse, but I was too frightened to walk into a police station without a comprehensive understanding of the process.

Not many people knew about the abuse and those who did only knew I'd *been abused* – not the details; keeping this secret was the only control I had over this terrible thing that had happened to me. I feared full disclosure because I feared handing control over to someone else. I feared the consequences of speaking out. I feared the abuser. Perhaps most of all I feared judgement. The shame was debilitating. This ISVA and I sat together for a couple of hours, and she asked me questions about what had happened. I tried but couldn't articulate it. I just couldn't say the right words – in fact, it was hard to say any words at all. The very word 'abuse' would get stuck somewhere between brain and mouth, and at times in the conversation I would be rendered completely mute.

At the end of our meeting, she said of course it was my choice whether or not to report it but that she would advise against it at this stage. She felt I wouldn't be able to withstand cross-examination if it got to trial. She asked me if I'd had specialist therapy for Child Sexual Abuse. I hadn't, so she put me on the two-year waiting list and referred me to a twelve-week 'self-confidence' course called The Way of The Goddess – a group for female survivors of sexual violence.

A few months later I found myself outside the building where the group was being held. It was at the end of my street, and I remember feeling mortified that I might be seen going to a support group and that I might be seen walking into the Samaritans. I wasn't sure what was worse – people thinking I was a survivor of sexual abuse or people thinking I was suicidal.

I was both.

New Year

To: Sophie Olson
From: Patricia Walsh
Hi Sophie,
Wishing you a Happy New Year and looking forward to meeting you soon.

You may well be feeling anxious about attending on the first day but remember that everyone you meet in the group will have gone through similar experiences and the course is especially designed for group clients and is not for attendance by members of the general public.

Groups are free. Tea, coffee, biscuits all provided. I will send an email with details of where to come etc and a little bit about the first session. Any questions meanwhile please do not hesitate to contact me.

If you are unable to attend, please notify me ASAP so that I can offer the place to another client as there is a waiting list.

Kind Regards,
Pat

Pat, who was facilitating the group, had said to call when I arrived so she could come down and let me in. I called the number with great trepidation and before long found myself on the top floor, in a group of eight women. Going into that room was perhaps one of the hardest – and with hindsight one of the most important steps I've ever taken. It was the very first step of my healing journey.

I had previous experience of group work and therapy in the Mental Health System – some good and some not so good. I had taken part in group rehab, attended Alcoholic Anonymous (AA), Narcotics Anonymous (NA) and therapy in a psychiatric hospital. I'd participated in group mindfulness, art, drama, CBT, yoga, psychotherapy, but these weren't groups specifically aimed at survivors. I appreciated being given time to draw and sculpt but none of the groups had helped me to speak about the Child Sexual Abuse. I entered this group on my guard – and one thing struck me immediately: every woman in the room had similar experiences to me.

It was unexpectedly comforting in that moment when I felt most uncomfortable to look at the other women and know they had experienced sexual violence, without even hearing them speak. They knew why I was there too. I'd never experienced this before; it was both liberating and overwhelming to see and be seen in this way.

My secrets were hidden from the outside world. The abused version of me – the *real me* as I perceived it – was like the smallest Russian doll, encased in layer after layer of carefully constructed other *me*s – acceptable versions of myself I presented to the rest of the world. I was a daughter – one layer. I was a wife – another layer. I was a mother of four children. I was a functioning, competent member of society – except I wasn't. These layers were a façade. The real me was trapped underneath. Silent and unseen in the dark – and this darkness was seeping through because the outer layers were cracking. These cracks were perceived as poor mental health, and some had seen the darkness underneath – the depression and suicidal ideation. People drew their own conclusions as to *why*, but they didn't care to look underneath this façade. If they had, they would have seen the shame. Under that they would have seen the fear, the silence, self-loathing and rage. Had they peeled that away, they would have seen the trauma of Child Sexual Abuse.

When I stepped into the freezing cold room on that grey, January morning, like everyone else I was announcing my abuse without having to say anything at all. It was as if these outer layers, the other *me*s, had been left at the door and it was disconcerting to know everyone could see the real version: the victim of Child Sexual Abuse. It made me feel exposed and vulnerable and I couldn't make eye contact with the others because the thought of seeing their pain made me feel deeply uneasy; I knew it would reflect my own. Part of me wanted to walk straight out of the room but another part was curious as to what would happen next.

I sat down choosing my escape route carefully – near the

door so I could leave with minimal disruption, and opposite the window so my mind could 'escape' if necessary – a skill I had developed as a child when physical escape wasn't possible. The group began. Some women were able to introduce themselves to the rest of the group and to divulge a bit of information, but other than saying my name, I stayed silent. I quickly realised with a surge of shame and a sinking heart that, as far as I knew, I was the only one with a background of non-recent sexual abuse. The other women in the group were survivors of adult domestic and sexual violence.

With hindsight, I realise there is nothing to say some of the women weren't abused in childhood too, but at the time the lack of reference to Child Sexual Abuse left me feeling angry and defensive. My abuse had been within my own family, and I was overwhelmed with shame. How would I be able to tell my story? What would they think of me? I stayed silent.

I contacted Pat afterwards demanding to know why I'd been referred to a group where I felt, yet again, different to everyone else. She encouraged me to come back the following week and said if I completed the course, an open-ended coffee morning would be available to me, where I would meet others with experience of non-recent and intrafamilial abuse. When I questioned why I couldn't skip the first group and move to the second group, she said I wouldn't be ready for it at that stage as the women were very open about their abuse, which could be overwhelming for me at this point.

I returned the following Tuesday and sat in my same spot by the door, still feeling cross, silent, and ashamed, but willing to try. I was to remain silent for a few weeks but as I listened to others tell their stories, I very slowly attempted to tell bits of my own.

Throughout the group sessions we were introduced to several written or drawing exercises, and about halfway through came one of the most important ones for both me and Pat. She gave us an outline of a mask to decorate, and this could be done in whatever way we chose, the aim being to illustrate the mask we wear day to day. Masks are a theme throughout the fairy tale because I presented a masked version of myself to the world, both as a young child and as an adult. It was an important activity as I felt able to communicate how locked away I was without having to speak the words. I slowly and methodically drew bricks until the mask was covered in a wall. This didn't feel enough so I drew bricks to cover my eyes and mouth. This was the first of many moments with Pat where I felt she understood what I was trying to say, despite being unable to say the words. By the time the twelve-week group came to an end, I was fully engaged with this concept of survivor community and pleased I had stuck with it, despite feeling challenged at times. I felt connected, for the first time in my life, to this incredible group of women, who just understood me. I was invited to join the coffee morning on a Tuesday morning.

My name is Patricia Walsh. I am an experiential and intuitive counsellor with over forty years' experience of working in trauma. This counselling approach allows me to work without judgement – to 'hear and listen', to 'see and gain insight' into the human being who has come to me for assistance.

I see my life experience as being equally as, if not more, important as my qualifications. Training provides education and knowledge and a way to evaluate that a certain standard of expertise has been reached. Life experience turns knowledge into wisdom. My first training to become a State Registered Nurse taught me caring and compassion, along with the importance of cleansing a wound diligently and deeply if it is going to heal. This technique I also apply to psychological wounds. My next training as an Occupational Therapist showed me the importance of engaging patients in purposeful activities, helping them to find a meaning to life when all seemed lost. My desire to explore the part that the mind plays in healing led me to train in Hypnotherapy and Psychotherapy at the National College of Hypnotherapy in London. This was followed by a BSc Hons in Psychology and a three-year training programme in Counselling & Psychotherapy to become a member of the National Counselling & Psychotherapy Society (NCPS). Throughout my studies, I was employed as an Independent Domestic Violence Advisor (IDVA) working with high-risk cases of domestic abuse. After qualifying as a counsellor, I was selected by the Police Firearms Officers Association for training in Trauma and PTSD. Recently, I have completed a course to become a Qigong practitioner. Using these techniques, I teach clients how to release trauma from the physical body and train the mind to become more resilient. It is also my own protective coping mechanism and allows me to work more efficiently with less chance of vicarious trauma.

Coffee Mornings

Spring – 12 Weeks Later

To: Pat
From: Sophie
Hello Pat,
    I just wanted to say sorry for having to rush off and also thank you very much for having me in your group. You are amazing to help so many women in the way that you do. I will do everything I can to make it to the coffee mornings.
    Sophie

To: Sophie
From: Pat
No problem. And it would be wonderful to see you there as you are getting ever closer to solving this yourself and I think the next sessions will help get you there.
    Take care.

To: Everyone
From: Pat
Hello everyone,
    Just a reminder about Tuesday.
    We are in the conference room on the second floor. Turn right at the top of the stairs, go through the door and past the red couch. Carry on forwards and you will find the conference room. Hope to see you there at 10 a.m.
    Pat

It was daunting to be starting the coffee morning group with new people and I greatly appreciated Pat's clear instructions on how to get to the room. Heightened anxiety of going to the wrong place could easily have prevented me from trying, and Pat's email showed she understood the challenges we might face, without drawing attention to it.

The coffee mornings were equally important as the previous group. There I met women further along on their journey than me, and they were to become my role models, leading by example. Seeing others reach the light, despite their trauma, despite most of them not receiving justice and feeling frustrated with the criminal justice system, gave me hope and encouragement that one day I might be able to heal too.

This hope was why I continued turning up each week, why I attended subsequent groups, and why I ultimately tried therapy again, even though it hadn't worked out for me previously.

At the first coffee morning I was overwhelmed by the honesty and conversations. I was both fascinated and appalled that women could freely speak about their own Child Sexual Abuse and their survival mechanisms. Pat being as astute as she always is, noticed my reaction and contacted me afterwards and these messages were the first time I alluded to my own suicidal ideation.

To: Sophie
From: Pat
Hi Sophie,
   Thank you for coming today. I am sure you found some of the stories these ladies had to tell very harrowing and upsetting and that is why it would have been hard for you to deal with in earlier days.
   Take care.
   Many thanks, Pat

To: Pat
From: Sophie
Hi Pat,
   Thank you.
   Yes, I found it a bit overwhelming today. There were so many faces. I'm not sure how to cope well today after the morning so maybe it's not right for me?

To: Sophie
From: Pat
I think only you can decide but by listening to all sides, you can start to decide, because as you heard today, there is no definite way to go forward and no perfect outcome. At the end of the day,

you know yourself better than anyone what you need to do to find an end to reliving the trauma and finding happiness.

To: Pat
From: Sophie
I don't know. I have no idea what to do to end this. Only one way for sure, which hurts my children. I just want to work and function as a normal person in society. I have to do this for my children but have never been able to live just for myself. I'm desperate to find a way.

To: Sophie
From: Pat
Hi Sophie,
   Go inside and begin to talk to the hurt and lonely child, just as if you were talking to your young children. Feel her needs and love her. When you can truly love her, then you will make peace with her, and you will live again. None of this was her fault so why blame her for someone else's sickness? I hope one day you will see the beauty radiating from you.

To: Pat
From: Sophie
Hi Pat,
   I would like to be able to do what you are doing, one day. To be able to help so many women is such an amazing thing. I'm glad I met you and discovered the groups. If it doesn't work out for me it is no reflection on the charity and the groups. Some people are unfortunately too broken to be put back together. I will try though.
   What I couldn't say in the group, was that it was because I felt shame. That's the biggest reason behind me not being able to voice any of this. Even naming the perpetrator in the group today was a huge step for me. I find it abhorrent and shameful that attempted rape makes me a survivor of CSA. I'm not sure why I'm telling you this – I know on an intellectual level that I don't need to feel this, but on an emotional level it is impossible for me not to at this stage.

'Attempted rape' was very deliberate phrasing.

The truth was far worse, but at this stage this was as far as I could go. I wanted to gauge Pat's reaction as well as try out a word I couldn't imagine verbalising. I waited for her to recoil in shock and horror.

To: Sophie
From: Pat
It's fine to say it to me ,Sophie, and I am so pleased you are now giving this horror a voice. Each time you say it, it becomes more real, and the extent of what he did to you will eventually turn to anger rather than shame. That's when you finally begin to feel again, and the anger turns to motivation and a will to live, rather than destroy. You are changing week by week, and it's wonderful to watch you opening like a beautiful flower deserving to be seen. You can come through this and turn not only your life but other people's lives around.
X

Had Pat not noticed my discomfort and used her intuition and reached out to me after this first session, I might not have returned to the next. Some might consider this an example of a professional crossing boundaries, but I view it differently. Pat opened a conversation where others might not have been courageous enough to do so.

I was at a crossroads. Should I continue or not?

The curiosity to see what would happen next, and the desire to hear more of these conversations spoken without fear or shame, surpassed my desire to check out of the world and I continued attending these coffee mornings every week, for the next couple of years.

A Small Taste of Activism

At one point I became instrumental in keeping the groups running. Funding cuts meant the room hire was no longer covered and I went on the hunt to find a new room. It was good practice for my future role in survivor activism. I banged on the doors of every church in a two-mile radius. I asked cafes, pubs, and local communities for the use of their halls and began to see first-hand the stigma surrounding CSA. This was particularly apparent in the response from churches. Some were happy to give us a free room for a 'women's group' but when they realised it was for survivors of CSA, they would come up with an excuse. *The room is taken after all . . . The elders don't think it's appropriate . . . - Our insurance won't cover you . . .* The Salvation Army was the one exception and because of their kindness, non-judgemental attitude and an indefinite offer of a room, free of charge, the coffee group was able to continue.

Funding then stopped for the twelve-week self-confidence courses and I was able to secure rooms for these too, at the local pub and then in a community hall. I went a step further and posted on a local Facebook group asking for donations of tea, coffee, and art supplies. Even though I wasn't outing myself as a survivor, it was the closest I'd come, and I hesitated before pressing 'post'. This Facebook group featured (not always friendly) discussions about parking and local wildlife. How would something like this be received? I was surprised by the replies. Some messaged me privately and a few disclosed their own experiences of abuse and asked if they could attend the group. It was the first time I recognised the power of speaking out.

To: Pat
From: Sophie
Hi Pat,
    I happen to know the vicar at *** Church. I'm determined to find a room! It's helping me too in a way because when I ask people, I'm also creating awareness and feeling more empowered

and less ashamed. Thank you for running the group today. It was helpful.

Sophie

It took a few more years before I was able to say I'd reached a point of 'recovery' (and I use that word *very* loosely, as I believe we learn to live alongside trauma rather than 'recover' from Child Sexual Abuse), and it required extensive therapy to get to that point. However, the validation, understanding and empathy I felt, simply by sitting in a room with other survivors played an important part of this journey. Feeling that sense of connection and being part of that community allowed me to form the support network I desperately needed. We needed each other and drew enormous strength from one another. Peer support was the first small step of a huge and treacherous mountain climb.

Two Steps Forward, One Step Back

Then I had a significant slip backwards. The specialist counselling I had been waiting for two years to access had finally come to fruition. I was in counselling with a woman I had begun to trust, when suddenly she moved on, out of the organisation. I had started my counselling with such hope to have finally found specialist support, so it was a devastating blow to be back at square one, to be told I would have to wait another two years. I was frightened by how fast this sense of hopelessness turned to suicidal ideation. The one person I trusted was Pat, the constant throughout these months of peer support, and I made a life-changing decision to reach out.

To: Pat
From: Sophie
Dear Pat,
 I'm sorry to bother you. I've lost all hope. I'm feeling like ending my life. I plan to do this as cleanly as possible and with no drama. I'm unable to see a way through. I could go to hospital I suppose, but I will only come back to this eventually. I'm unwell. My children are seeing this sickness in me, and they have the right to live peacefully without this. Once they grieve then life can move on for them. It will be hard, but they have each other. Thank you for everything. You have been a wonderful support. I think I found you too late in life.
 X

To: Sophie
From: Pat
Sophie,
 I have only just picked up your message. I've tried to phone you but no reply. Can you get back to me tonight if possible.
No one can replace a mother. It is so devastating for children.

To: Sophie
From: Pat
Sophie,
    I hope you have decided not to do what you planned. I have tried phoning. I hope your family is supporting you until you can get help.

To: Pat
From: Sophie
Please don't worry about phoning me or contacting me as I don't want to worry anyone. It is preying very heavily on my mind at the moment, and it was important to me to thank you but I'm not asking for your help.

To: Sophie
From: Pat
Dear Sophie,
    Thank you for getting back to me. I really appreciate it. When you get low to this point again, think how you would feel if one of your children were to take their own life – you would be devastated. We all matter to each other because we are all connected. I didn't realise how much I mattered to my sons, until I was slowly dying, and I decided to come back for that reason. I'm very glad that I did, because the best was yet to come.

To: Pat
From: Sophie
Were you depressed?
    I'm sorry. I shouldn't have asked. It's none of my business.

To: Sophie
From: Pat
It's fine, it might just help you. I am currently writing about the group work practice and how I came to it through my own personal journey. I think it is time for me to capture what happens when you come out the other side of life's difficulties.

To: Pat
From: Sophie
Pat,
I don't think I can hang on. I'm so frightened. My husband thinks I need to be in hospital.

To: Sophie
From: Pat
What do you think?
I would ask you why you hate yourself for something someone else did when you were so young and vulnerable. I also suspect you are not the only one. By hating yourself you are taking the blame for someone else's inhumane behaviour.
   Depression is anger turned inwards, so let the anger out, but not in the form of self-destruction, and when the anger does come, ask yourself what do you want to do with it to change it from harming you?

To: Pat
From: Sophie
I'm angry outwardly too. I can't trust myself to drive. I don't hate myself. I just don't wish to live like this anymore. I'm tired and I've had enough. I had more children so they would have each other. This was always in the cards for me. Much as I liked to pretend I was living a normal life, I wasn't.
   I'm scared of dying and don't seem to be very good at it. I'm scared of living like this though as well. You think this is new for me because you haven't known me for long, but I have been like this before, and I have been angry and agitated. Speaking about the abuse is the only difference really. My consultant diagnosed me with bipolar 2 disorder but the side effects from the medications are so awful. I know tomorrow she will try to put me on medication, but the side effect can be hair loss, which I'm not prepared to risk. I'm running out of options.

To: Sophie
From: Pat
The only option is to dare. Dare to go out and live. Live as if you are having the dance of your life. When you have done that, you will no longer be afraid to die, because you will know that you have come here to do what you were meant to do.

You are not his abuse, he is.

You are not the past; you are the here and now with the future ahead.

Decide what you want to do with the anger. Either shop him and get past the fear, or don't shop him and decide to put it to rest – only you can decide. If you decide nothing, it is like deliberately standing under a crumbling brick wall and letting fate decide. Make a move and things will fall into place. You say you are tired of living like this, that you have had enough. Removing yourself from this life to release this tiredness might feel like it's all you can do right now, but when there are others involved, sometimes you have to take that into consideration. Instead, imagine for a moment how it would be if you turned it all around for your children. What a role model they would have!

That could be you if you chose it, and it would mean so much for others too. Imagine one day being a spokeswoman for all of this, or a member of parliament – you have the contacts! How scary would that be for him?

To: Pat
From: Sophie
That all sounds good but I haven't got any idea how to do that. I'd love to DO something. Finding the room was doing something but that's done. I have no relevant qualification, no degree. No one could possibly take me seriously. I think maybe in a parallel life I am doing these things. I'm sorry. You are saying kind things and you are very supportive, but I think it's not going to happen because I don't know where to begin. I haven't been employed for so long and I have no confidence in my ability.

I was going to ask you to give up on me but I don't think you give up on people often.

To: Sophie
From: Pat
No, it's not part of my remit. Giving up is not an option because everyone matters. I can only reach the group for as long as the group runs but you will all in turn touch each other's lives, and care for each other.

Safeguarding

As a Member of the National Counselling and Psychotherapy Society (NCPS), I carried out Sophie's safeguarding according to their Code of Ethics, which states that all practitioners undertake to:

> 'Maintain strict confidentiality within the client/counsellor relationship, always provided that such confidentiality is neither inconsistent with the therapist's own safety or the safety of the client, the client's family members or other members of the public, nor in contravention of any legal action (i.e., criminal, coroner or civil court cases where a court order is made demanding disclosure) or legal requirement (e.g., Children's Acts).'

The NCPS elaborates further by stating that working with clients who are at risk of suicide or serious self-harm creates an immensely challenging situation for the therapist because in British Law there is no duty to rescue. Therapists need to be explicit with clients about reserving the power to breach confidentiality for a suicidal adult client. To breach without explicit agreement may constitute an actionable breach of confidence. If a therapist knows that a client is likely to harm themselves or others but will not give their consent for referral, then careful consideration must be given to the ethics of going against the client's known wishes and the possible consequences for the client in the therapist making a referral or not doing so.

Throughout Sophie's therapy, self-harm and suicidal ideation were a constant challenge and a live risk as these two options had been her ultimate default coping mechanism as an adult.

As her therapist, my management of this situation is cited in the chapter *Two Steps Forward, One Step Back*, in which Sophie first talks to me about suicide. I suggested family involvement and the possibility of accessing other interventions. We opened a dialogue on suicide and depression, allowing verbalisation and validation of her feelings. The importance of this is shown later, when Sophie comments on the role that dialogue and support, particularly quick responses, feeling safe and being held, had had for her sense of wellbeing.

Throughout her therapy with me, Sophie spoke a lot about the possible consequences of her being admitted to a psychiatric hospital. Her experiences of hospital became a benchmark for my choices around her safeguarding. It was obvious that autonomy was critically important for her.

However, as illustrated later in the chapter *I Don't See the Point to this Anymore*, while appreciating Sophie's innate ability to make her own decisions, I strongly recommended to her that her intuition about not feeling safe should be listened to, and any thoughts that her husband and family had about her needing to go to hospital should be given serious consideration as a preferred course of action. In a later chapter, I also recommended that Sophie engaged the help of her previous psychiatrist with whom she had established a good rapport. Sophie did this by emailing her. At one point, with Sophie's permission, when she had left home in a highly distressed state, I called her husband, telling him where she was. He collected her and elected to take her home, rather than call the mental health crisis team. During this time of crisis, I remained on the phone talking to her until I knew that her husband had reached her.

At this point in time, there were two major contributing factors to Sophie's experience of crisis. Firstly, although her husband was aware of her therapy, she had never revealed to him her level of self-harming, neither in the past nor the present, or the extent of the Child Sexual Abuse she had endured. She was revealing this, to me, for the first time. At each stage of her revelation, she was waiting for me to reject her.

Secondly, there was the connection to Sophie's physical health, and this contributed to the reduction of her resilience. As you will see in the following chapters, Sophie's physical health is entwined with her trauma. At the time of this crisis, Sophie had taken on excessive sewing orders that were beyond what she could physically manage. Given the fact that Sophie ordinarily experiences high levels of back pain, the pain was now so exacerbated that her prescribed analgesia could no longer alleviate it.

Ultimately, when a person reaches the state of entering the dark abyss – the place of suicide – all a therapist can do, or indeed all anyone can do, is hold a light for them, take their hand and guide them back onto the path. It was at this point that Sophie finally realised that she was the only one who held the answer to her survival.

Therapy with Pat Begins

Autumn

To: Pat
From: Sophie
Hi Pat,
　Please can you let me know if you have any space for private therapy or if there is a waiting list?
　Thank you.
　Sophie

To: Sophie
From: Pat
You are welcome to try a trial session with me. You would need to think out what you want from your counselling. There is no pressure, and ultimately you have to feel comfortable.

To: Pat
From: Sophie
Please could we start with the trial session and then take it from there?

To: Sophie
From: Pat
That's fine. I will book you in and see what you want to do. We can treat it more like an introductory session of chatting about your expectations for counselling and what more you feel you need. I will give you time to think about it before you sign paperwork, etc. In my private counselling, if I take notes, I give them to the client in a folder to take away with them. The client brings them back the next week and can decide if they want to discuss anything that arises from the notes any further. We add to the notes as we go. The only notes I keep outside of this is a record of attendance and a few headings of the topics we discussed.

I felt very lucky to have crossed paths with such an intuitive therapist and that Pat was able to become mine. She has helped many like me. It shouldn't be so hard to access this sort of support and yet it is. At the first face to face session, I handed her a written broad outline of the abuse. The focus was on the emotional abuse because I was unable, at this stage, to go into detail about the sexual abuse.

~ Sophie
Thank you for the session, Pat. It may sound like a strange request, but please can you let me know when you've read what I left with you? I feel like I've handed over my soul.

~ Pat
I will read it tonight after my sessions have finished here and text you.

Sophie, sorry for the delay. I have just got home and read what you have written. No wonder you feel you have handed over your soul to me. You have entrusted to me the fragments of your soul – a soul that needs restoring and I hope I can help you do that. You are one of the most amazing human beings I have ever come across and your survival is even more astonishing. What you showed me before shocked me. What you have given me now, there are no words to describe. I have underlined some things that are particularly relevant to what we spoke about today so we will look at this together next time. Thank you for sharing this with me. It has helped to increase my understanding further. Take care and see you soon.

Is it too much? It's left me feeling that I've overshared, which is stupid as that's what you're there for.

There is no question of oversharing. I am here as your listener and for you to give voice to these atrocities which have been your inner world for too long. Thankfully, Sophie, I am blessed with a way to deal with people's trauma so that it does not become my own, so do not be concerned for me. Take care of yourself and enjoy your weekend.

OK. Thank you.

Winter

Hello, I'm so sorry to contact you during the holidays. I'm having a tough couple of days of flashbacks and struggling a bit with it. I needed to touch base with you. I hope you had a good Christmas x

Hi Sophie, would you like a call later? Write the flashbacks down to remind yourself they are all in the past. As you write each flashback down, name the emotions that go with the visuals to help you validate them. Remember to let go of the breath and exhale forcefully through your mouth, so your lungs are helping to release the stored trauma. You might also need your little dog for emotional warmth and comfort, so snuggle up.

I don't need a call, thank you. I'm not great at speaking on the phone. Just messaging you helps and makes me feel less alone. I can't talk to anyone else around me.

No problem at all. Keep messaging me. These flashbacks are showing you that the mind is prepared to let them be seen. If you can, then let them play out . . . this happened and then this and then this, until they are done. Then write them down, name what happened and remind yourself that you were living with a very, very, sick dead-eyed person and not all the world is like that . . . You have a lovely husband and children and you have survived.

Not all flashbacks are real though. The dreams at night are a warped and distorted version. I'm writing them down.

No, they may not all be real, but they are trying to give a reality to what happened. Your dream of the staircase [shared in a face-to-face session] and not being able to see the face of the woman and there being no safety – that revealed a lot as you explored it with me.

The dreams are focusing on the house and on Wednesday I'm going back there for a family gathering. We will be mainly in

the room that was most unsafe. I have a choice not to go of course, but it's not that simple unfortunately.

Yes, you do have a choice. Think very carefully about it because you are no longer the child without any choices. You can now do exactly what you want. On the other hand, if you feel you must go, use it as part of your therapy. Remind yourself this was in the past . . . that this person can no longer harm you . . . What do you want to say about this house and the room and to whom? If you could get any sort of justice for what happened there, what would that be? What does the adult Sophie need to do to take charge of being made to revisit this house? Finally, what does the adult Sophie want to say to the little child who suffered so badly in that house?

I feel that I'm beginning to recall more. They're not all memories as such, they're frustratingly out of reach, but they are very intense feelings. I don't know what to trust as real.

Don't worry right now about what is real and unreal. Just go with the emotions because they hold the key to the memories. It is intense emotions that lock down the memory . . . The good thing is the adult is starting to take control in the dreams you are having, as if gradually guiding the child. Just allow yourself to trust you.

I'm drawing non-stop. It's helpful to draw what I remember but some are so awful, I have to rip them up and throw them away.

Try not to throw them – put them in a folder and bring them to me.

If I'm not ready to do it, where do we go then, next week?

Next week we can explore feelings, both then and now. At any time, you can have a break. This is your path to recovery, and you should feel in charge of it. I am there to listen and guide. The more you are processing, the more suppressed memories will emerge because the unconscious will realise a safety net is being created and that no retrieved memory can be as bad as what you have already physically experienced and survived.

We haven't discussed how long I will see you for. Is there a set amount of time you like to work with clients, or do we play it by ear?

Play it by ear – sometimes taking sessions to fortnightly and then monthly, as it all begins to come together for you.

I think it could be helpful for you to be able to see my board on Pinterest. Like my drawings, I selected images in a bit of a trance-like state, some of them without thinking much about it but feeling strong emotion when viewing it.

Yes, it would be good if you could share these images with me. Even if you could send them individually that would be helpful, as I could then put them together in a folder. It is the emotions with visuals that help release memories. They can then be given language. It is the emotions that numb us, when it becomes too painful to feel anymore. Once we get an emotion, we can go to where you are feeling this, and ask questions such as, does it have a colour, etc?

When I couldn't speak the words I needed to say; when I was mute with shame, habit and fear, Pat came up with alternative approaches. Pat told me of other women who had found creative ways to express the horrors, such as the creation of a doll's house, a Japanese Zen garden, painting, collage or drawing. We tried different things and each one unlocked another bolt to a 'Big Black Door' – a visual barrier in my mind behind which I pushed the memory of trauma. When flashbacks of images, memories of sound and sensations of touch, taste or smell came to the forefront, I moved them to the back, behind this imagined door that I pictured locking and bolting. It was a successful method but only up to a point.

Pinterest was a useful tool. I made a secret board of images, about one hundred in total. Photographs of a cuff or a watch on a man's wrist. 1980s decor. A tumbler of whisky. A child's pair of red Wellington boots. An escalator. A chicken coop. Each image had a story and they all needed to be told but I wasn't sure how to, so I printed the images and, in a session, laid them out in a timeline and divided this timeline into different ages: up to four years old, four to seven, seven to nine and nine to ten.

Later I would talk about being fourteen, but that memory I didn't process until later.

> **Thank you for looking at them. It was harder than I thought to share them. I think they give me something to work on with you though.**

> They do. I can start to intuitively work with them as I familiarise myself with the picture and what you have called them, because I will name each one as I store it. Pictures and drawings are such a useful way of working. They make contact with our emotions, and the adult self can begin to integrate with the lost child.

> **My hair pulling is out of control. I'll be bald when I see you next. Seriously.**

> Time to stop, Sophie, on these pictures and have a break. Ask yourself what else you can use instead of this destructive coping mechanism. Ask the adult because this is the child's old coping mechanism. Maybe time to find a new creative crochet product for spring?

> **I'm not usually aware I'm doing it until I've been doing it for a while, when I kind of come to and see the hair that I've pulled out, then I try and stop it. But I will stop the pictures now.**

> Can you do something with that patch of hair, such as put a small pretty hair grip there to remind you not to pull it?

> **It's my whole head. I run my fingers through until a hair catches and pulls out. Sometimes it helps if I tie it back.**

> Then maybe tie it back while you are working on these things.

I sent more images to Pat.

> I will work on these over the weekend and file them into folders. At least I have them now and can study and reflect on them.

Will we use them tomorrow?

> Yes, we can if you would like to.

I've been unable to look at my drawing. I need to do that with you, I think.

> That's fine we'll take it at your pace and what you can manage. You have come so far.

Have I? It doesn't feel like it at the moment.

> A few weeks ago, you hadn't even drawn pictures or put these photos together.

Behind the Big Black Door

Following the next session, I sent Pat more pictures and then made the difficult decision to visit a place where I remembered being taken to by the abuser as a child. A few of my memories of sexual abuse, especially from the occasions where it happened outside of the house, were incomplete and this frustrated me. I thought I needed to remember *everything* to start recovering from the trauma.

> **Hi Pat, I'm sitting in the lay-by and feeling so bloody frustrated because I just can't remember. I need to retrieve the memories. I need to remember everything that happened to my body in that car, and I can't. I feel like throwing up and my heart is racing but the memory isn't there.**
>
> Then just leave it be. Perhaps if we work through more pictures first, because probably the car episode may prove to be the most traumatic of all.
>
> **It's so frustrating. I feel like I don't have control of my own brain.**
>
> Generally, we have no memories of out of body experiences because the trauma has been too great for us to cope with . . .
>
> Let this just gradually flow and begin with the drawings you can manage to look at and explain to me. This will gradually become acceptable to the unconscious as it then passes into conscious memories and becomes processed.
>
> **But isn't it also normal for people who haven't experienced trauma to not remember parts of childhood?**
>
> It can happen if there are parts that are not very interesting but why would the lay-by keep coming back to you so powerfully

if there was nothing to explore? Also, out of body experiences are not normal in young children unless trauma is involved.

Going there left me with the strong urge to self-harm. I keep visualising it.

So now you know that this part is not available to you for a reason. You have to wait until you are ready. Remember always, when you feel overwhelmed, this is not your stuff and he should never have been anywhere near children – he is a very, very sick person.

I am ready. I haven't acted upon the urge, and I don't think I will. Old habits die hard.

The old habits are old, conditioned responses, and now we are looking at new . . . to get to grips with his dark stuff and for you to live your life to the full and shine like the beautiful person you are.

But you're wrong about it not being my stuff. He made it mine as it was my body. Self-harm is a way of purging that.

Regarding the stuff being yours, when you were the child you had no choice, but as the adult you do. He tried to take your mind, as well as your body, but couldn't and for those who survive, it is our job to transform this dark into light, so that it no longer harms us or those around us.

Then we tried art. When an inpatient in a psychiatric hospital ten years earlier, I had drawn constantly and they were repetitive images of figures, many in the same position with one arm over the face. Although I didn't share these with Pat until later, I started to draw again, this time to express what I couldn't say. Each session unlocked another bolt to the Big Black Door, but I felt helpless because I still couldn't speak the words, and I wanted Pat to read my mind. What if I could never say the actual words and they stayed inside me forever, infecting, festering, and making my body and mind sick?

> Therapeutically, Sophie's drawings and Pinterest board were as important to understanding her as the mask of bricks had been in our earlier work together during the group sessions. Her drawings were releasing her unconscious mind, sometimes in a way far more powerfully than words. They are the most ancient form of human expression and yet understood universally in their simplicity. The mask of bricks covered the whole of Sophie's face including her eyes and mouth. It was as challenging for me as it was for her. 'How will you make me speak? How will you make me see again? How will you build trust with me to see what is inside this mask and when you do . . . what then?
>
> [See Picture One – Mask of Bricks.]

Pat made the decision to free up the next hour after my sessions to allow me time to speak some of the toxic, poisonous words that sat under the surface. She could see they were ready to spill over, but my courage to speak was usually found ten minutes before the end. Pat didn't tell me *time's up* or *see you next week*. She told me to *forget time*, that this was *much more important than time*. Having this extra hour made all the difference to me.

Telling our stories and processing trauma is hard work – risky at times and, for me, the flashbacks increased. The last time I'd experienced flashbacks to that extent was the day my daughter turned nine, when I had looked at her and seen myself as the child victim of rape. Those flashbacks led to a suicide attempt that ended up in a long hospitalisation.

When I started to tell my story to Pat, I felt myself being pulled once more into the abyss. This made me angry and frustrated because therapy seemed to be making me WORSE not better. If this is what happened when you tried to heal yourself then what was the point? How could I process this AND continue functioning as a mother? How could I ride nights of broken sleep and night terrors and then take my children to school? How could I do household chores or remember to practice spelling tests, write a shopping list, or walk the dog when I could feel physical sensations of abuse?

I felt the familiar, old feelings of despair settling in my heart. This was impossible. I would never be free from abuse. The shadows came back and filled my head. I began to think suicide was part of my destiny. Perhaps it always had been, and I was just delaying the inevitable.

When I voiced these thoughts to Pat, shame enveloped me, weighing me down in a heavy blanket. I waited to be told – as I had been by a psychiatrist and other mental health professionals in the past – that these thoughts were selfish, that indeed I was selfish to consider such an act as a mother of four children.

When mental health professionals respond in this way to a mother who is at breaking point, they may do so with good intentions, but deep down they must realise it's a way of shutting that person down. It's rewarding the excruciating and risky baring of one's soul with judgement and cruelty. Their words cut like a knife. Our hearts bleed and we might not reach out for help again.

In my opinion, society tells CSA survivors *they* are the problem. Desperate acts of survival in a world where there is no outlet for this type of trauma are considered symptomatic of illness. *These things you're doing to yourself – do you think that's normal? You need treatment, medication, perhaps an inpatient stay.* But many of us will feel there is no other choice, having sensed from childhood the reluctance to hear our stories. This message is reinforced by the mental health system. We are told to *try making a cup of tea*, or to *take a warm bath*. We are told to *snap an elastic band* on our wrists when we need to self-harm. It is seemingly fine to hurt ourselves as long as we do it in a way that doesn't impinge on others. As long as our anguish is not *too* visible.

Pat didn't tell me I was selfish. She reminded me that my children needed a mother but not in a way that shamed or silenced. She didn't seem surprised or horrified. She didn't call my GP or suggest I go to A & E. She answered in her usual calm and unperturbed way: 'You know deep down psychiatrists, me, medication, harming . . . none have the answer. The only answer is to find a depth of strength within you to survive through this.'

I kept surviving. I got up each day, I took my children to school, and I existed, functioned, but barely. I took it one day, hour, sometimes a minute at a time. Pat made it clear through her quick responses to my messages that she was there for me. Knowing that there was someone at the other end of the phone was a lifeline and I felt safe and held in a way I hadn't experienced before. Without this level of support, or if I'd been admitted to a psychiatric hospital at this point, I doubt I would have carried on with the therapy. I would have been back at square one, or I would have died.

Try Writing It as a Fairy Tale

Spring

And then came the session where I felt I would give up. I felt frustrated, as I'd worked so hard on trying to speak but the most important words; the worst ones, had simply not come out. I implied I would not necessarily come back the following week and as I got up to leave the room, Pat said, 'Try detaching from it entirely. Try writing it as a fairy story. Start with the words: once upon a time there was a little girl.'

That evening, I tried. I sat on my bed and typed on the Notes app of my phone *Once Upon A Time* . . . and finally, four decades after the abuse began, the words started to flow.

After about twenty minutes I had the first chapter sitting in my hands. The process of writing had been a cathartic release, yet it felt dangerous, like a loaded bomb. I wasn't sure what to do next. My body fired with the distressing physical memory of abuse. My heart ached. My head was full of images I'd spent my life pushing away and shutting down. I messaged Pat, not expecting an answer as it was late at night but, again, this amazing woman was there for me.

It is risky to be honest when we feel we're losing our grip on sanity. In my first message I describe myself as 'struggling a little'. In reality, I was in a state of terror and was tipping into a state of crisis. These messages grounded me and without them my story would have been very different.

> Sorry to message you. Is it OK? I've been really fine, now I'm struggling a little.

> Of course, you can message me. It was a difficult session for you. Be really easy on yourself. You are a very brave woman

in confronting this, and trying to make sense of the state of that poor little girl is very difficult – it's as bad as what you went through.

I can feel him.

So, keep talking to your body. He is no longer here. This is not happening now, and keep shaking down from your body . . .start to belly-breathe lying on your back. Fill your belly up like a baby does, like a balloon and place your hands over that area so you are comforted by the rise and fall of your abdomen. Then put yourself into your trance-like state and take your mind back to being the baby in the womb before this all happened and allow yourself to rest in the stillness. It's the place where we call the void . . .it's a place of deep peace and stillness. I think I showed you this exercise.

Yes, you have. It helps at the time. Then it comes back again. I'm writing it away too.

Brilliant . . . keep on releasing it until it's done for a while . . . Tell yourself with that amazing mind of yours that you no longer need to carry this stuff. I am studying with someone currently who knows about trauma release and the physical somatisation of memories. Any techniques I can glean, I will send them over.

Can I send my writing over to you? I need to do something with it.

Yes, do, that's not a problem at all. I will pick it up in a little while.

And here it is. The first chapter of my life. I sent it to Pat and the feeling of that is hard to describe. Disclosure is akin to detonating the bomb. What would happen next? Would she react in a way that validated my shame or validated my experiences? What would she think of me? How could I look her in the eye next time we met? Perhaps most importantly of all, would she believe me?

Chapter 1

The Kingdom of His

'Come with me,' the swallow said, after Thumbelina had made a hole in the tunnel roof. 'If you sit on my wings, I will take you to the green forest and the sun will kiss your pretty hair.'

– Thumbelina, Hans Christian Andersen

Once upon a time, at the top of a hill, in the middle of an island, sat a pretty cottage with pink roses around the door. The cottage was surrounded by high walls built by the Evil King to keep out the rest of The World.

The Evil King was very powerful. He was tall, strong, clever and rich and wore clothes made from the finest fabrics.

Every day he patrolled the gardens, checking the high walls for gaps. He carried wood and nails and would *tap, tap, tap* his way around the garden until he was satisfied that no prying eyes could see inside his kingdom.

He named his kingdom His.

A Little Princess lived inside The Kingdom of His. She had blonde hair and brown eyes, but her clothes were made from rags and scraps. The Evil King wanted the finest things for himself as he needed to show The World how powerful, strong and clever he was.

The Little Princess was a sad princess. She knew of this place called The World, because the Evil King sometimes took her out with him. He would dress the Little Princess in pretty clothes and brush her hair. Then he would open a box and remove two Masks that he kept especially for these journeys to The World. The large Mask was a Kind and Gentle Mask.

This Mask, the Evil King put on his own face. It covered up the Ugliness and Evil underneath. The smaller Mask was a Happy Mask. He put this one on the Little Princess. This Mask covered up the sadness that the Evil King didn't want The World to see. The Evil King would then pick up the Little Princess and carry her through The World. When he saw people looking, he would pretend to laugh and play with the Little Princess. He pretended to the people who lived in The World that he was a kind and gentle king and they all wanted to be his friend and thought the Little Princess a lucky princess. They showered him with gifts and money because they loved him so much and he used it to buy more fine clothes for himself and more wood and nails for the high walls.

The Little Princess liked seeing The World, but it made her feel empty inside. She knew she could never be part of The World as her place was in The Kingdom of His.

When they returned home, the Evil King would remove their Masks one by one and place them carefully in the box. He locked them away in a cupboard where they stayed until next time. He removed the Little Princess's pretty clothes and dressed her in rags and scraps.

The Little Princess wished he would laugh and play again but when she tried to make him laugh and play, he looked at her with his pale blue eyes and she knew she was in great danger. His eyes were made of Cold Ice and when he looked at her, they turned her into a Frozen Statue. She wanted to run away but she couldn't. The Little Princess's legs and arms became cold, heavy and Useless. When she tried to lift them, they stayed frozen to the spot. She only melted when he looked away. She didn't like being a Frozen Statue so she learned not to look at his Cold Ice Eyes and to stay as far away from him in the cottage as she could.

* * *

One day, when the Little Princess was lying in her bed, the Evil King came to her and started to laugh and play. *That's strange,* thought the Little Princess, *why is he laughing and playing when there is no one else from The World to see?*

She glanced to see if he was wearing his Mask, but he wasn't.

The Ugliness was there for her to see and the Little Princess was confused. *Maybe I am mistaken,* she thought to herself. *Maybe he doesn't need a Mask because he is kind and gentle after all?*

The Little Princess decided to look at his eyes to find out for sure, but then a terrible thing happened. The Ice in the Evil King's eyes hadn't melted at all. They were colder and harder than ever and when her brown eyes saw the Ice, in an instant she was frozen to her bed and the Little Princess started to shrink. She got smaller and smaller until she feared she would disappear completely.

The Evil King stopped laughing and playing and he held the tiny, frozen Princess in his Evil hands. The Little Princess tried in vain to move her body, but she couldn't. She was caught in a trap.

The Little Princess felt something crawling on her Body and she saw the Evil King's fingers had turned into Snakes. Ten, twenty, a hundred, one thousand writhing Snakes began to crawl over the Little Princess. They crawled under her clothes and into her hair. They crawled up her legs and wrapped themselves around her arms. When they began to crawl into her mouth, the Little Princess knew she would die if she didn't escape.

But what can I do? thought the Little Princess. *Surely, I will die because I am frozen to my bed and can't escape.*

Although the Little Princess's Body didn't work, her ears could hear, and her eyes could see.

Come here, come with us, she heard, and she looked out of the window. Little birds sat on the windowsill. *Come with us,* they said, *fly away, fly away.*

And the Little Princess found that she didn't need her Body after all and that she could fly away using her eyes. Following the birds, the Little Princess rose from the bed, and leaving her Body to the Snakes, floated away, away, out of the cottage, over the high walls and into The World where the sun shone brightly and the sky was blue.

Exploring 'The Kingdom of His'

Pat responded to me within half an hour.

To: Sophie
From: Pat
This is so expressive and eventually when you are ready, it should be shared with others. Thank God or whatever that you had the ability to go out of body because that way he could not destroy your beautiful mind. That is why, dear Sophie, you have no clear memories of what he did because if you did, you would no longer be here. Such a beautiful princess and such a sick, horrific monster, unable to feel anything for others. Take care and well done you. You are truly amazing, and I am honoured to be working with someone so truly wonderful and special.

To: Pat
From: Sophie
I have got memories. I didn't always do this. I feel sick to my stomach. Thank you so much. That's a lovely thing to say. Thank you x.

To: Sophie
From: Pat
It is so time now to live, Sophie, for you, your lovely husband, and your beautiful children.

It is worth noting the time of night I sent this first chapter, and that Pat replied to me – 11pm. I often wonder what I would have done if she hadn't replied. Would my shame have pushed me to breaking point? Sending this was the closest I'd got to saying what had actually happened. I could still only do so in this abstract fairy tale format, but if she hadn't replied, I don't think I would have been able to go back the next week to my appointment. It would have been another failed attempt at therapy.

    I said, *I have got memories. I didn't always do this.* It was important that Pat didn't think my memories were recovered. I grew up in the 1990s during a time when false memory syndrome made headline news. One of my fears was being accused of retrieving false memory or of being told they were implanted through the process of therapy. What I didn't understand then was that memory can be both clear and fragmented. Despite clear memories of abuse, I feared the fragments. Later, one of the most fragmented memories of all would be written into a chapter called *The Basement* and the courage to write that came after speaking with my family who were able to confirm that the clear memory – the room I remembered being taken to – did exist.

I needed a lot of validation from Pat. I had spent years hiding my trauma and put significant effort into hiding the consequences of trauma on the adult I had become. As well as this fear of being disbelieved, I worried people might gaslight my recall of events or minimise the trauma in the way I had minimised it – *Oh, it's not that bad. I got over it. Other people experience worse.* To start processing it, I needed someone to tell me it was worthy of being processed.

Because of Pat's response, I felt able to keep writing. Some may critcise her for describing him as a 'sick, horrific monster', but it's hard to express quite *how much* I needed someone else to say that. No one ever had and it felt like she *just got it*. I pictured her standing by my side as we faced the Big Black Door and together sliding back a bolt. As you will read later on, this door had opened in the past, but it had been violently blown open and nobody had been able to help me contain the memories that had overwhelmed me – leaving me in a highly vulnerable state. Pat, and her response to this first and most important chapter, made me feel safe and so I continued, sending her the next chapter I called *The Old Witch*, which describes my earliest memory of self-harm.

Chapter 2

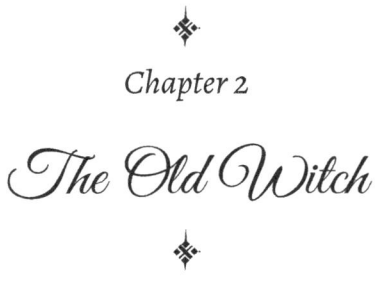

'As soon as they have you in their power they will kill you without mercy, and cook and eat you, for they are eaters of men. If I did not take pity on you and save you, you would be lost.'

– The Robber Bridegroom, The Brothers *Grimm*

Princess!

The Old Witch loudly shouted from somewhere inside the Little Princess and it woke her up. The Little Princess wondered where she had been and why she had to come back. She remembered birdsong and blue sky but now she was on her own, in her bedroom, in the cottage, within the high walls, far away from The World.

The Little Princess couldn't see the Old Witch, but she could hear her now, as she grumbled and cursed. Her bemoaning voice annoyed the Little Princess. The Little Princess wanted to leave with the birds again, but every time she tried, the Old Witch would shout and distract the Little Princess. She didn't want to be in the cottage, and she didn't want to have her Body back. The Little Princess decided she didn't like her Body anymore. It was Weak and Stupid. It didn't do what she asked it to do. It hurt to have a Body.

The Little Princess wondered if she could punish her Body, like the way she was sometimes punished by the Evil King.

She lifted her skirts, and hit and punched her legs.

Grumble, grumble, went the Old Witch.

The Little Princess hit and punched and hit and punched until the blood rose to the surface, ready to spill. But her fists were too small and Useless, so she looked for a hairbrush and hit and hit and hit with the bristles, until the blood flowed.

The Little Princess was glad.

'Useless stupid Body,' she said.

The Little Princess punished The Body every time she remembered The Snakes.

'It's your fault,' she said. 'You didn't run away.' She hit as hard as she could and the pain from the hitting and punching stopped the Little Princess from remembering the crawling of The Snakes. The Little Princess felt the pain in her Body from The Snakes. They had crushed and bitten the Little Princess and she felt angry with her Body for letting them hurt her.

She searched and searched in the cottage until she found a magic potion to heal the Snake bites. She discovered that soothing her Body made her dislike it more than ever. Even so, she carefully hid the magic potion, just in case The Snakes came back.

And the Old Witch grumbled.

Exploring 'The Old Witch'

To: Sophie
From: Pat
This is a complete insight into self-harming and why someone would do this. It would be so powerful to use this to explain to teachers, parents, and health professionals about what happens for a small child when faced with such a horrific nightmare. Thank you so much for sharing.

To: Pat
From: Sophie
It's about anger and frustration, isn't it? If you feel powerless, you feel weak and that it's your fault, or your body's fault, for being unable to do the things you need it to do. You are too small, too insignificant and there is a dichotomy between this and the adult war that these children are experiencing and surviving.

To: Sophie
From: Pat
Yes, that's right – you are absolutely correct. Also, your emotions become numb and your heart closes because it becomes too painful to feel anymore. Self-harming allows you to feel physical pain even more, and it allows you to feel again, but in a destructive way.

How to explain the Old Witch? As a young child I sometimes heard a voice inside my head. It sounded like an old woman, and I pictured her as a crone – a witch that grumbled away in the background. I knew only I could hear her, and that didn't concern me, and she didn't concern me either, but I viewed her as an inconvenience as I found her distracting at times. Sometimes I heard her shout my name and I would 'come back' from wherever I was inside my head. Other than that, I never made out distinct words but her overall tone was one of displeasure and criticism. The first time I self-harmed as a child, she was there. I decided to write about her and send it to Pat because I believed she was connected to abuse. I'm sure psychologists will have their own take on what exactly was going on but now I view her as an instinct, perhaps my own inner voice, that I had to suppress as a child.

Children who are sexually abused by those in a position of trust, by someone they know, have no choice but to suppress their instinct in order to survive. They might hear the words *I love you* as they cuddle up for a bedtime story with an abuser. CSA is not always violent. It doesn't always happen in secret places. It happens in children's beds, at bedtime, bath-time, in the kitchen, on the way to school and is often enmeshed with normality. One hand turning the page of a favourite story and the other creeping up the thigh. It is confusing for that child to receive constant mixed messages. They begin to detach from the inner voice and override instinct in order to survive the abuse. They start to wonder, *Why, when you tell me you love me, do you hurt me?* But there are no answers.

Hurt and love begin to mean the same thing, which makes us vulnerable to being hurt again in future relationships as we navigate life. It is not unusual for survivors of sexual abuse to suffer further abuse and, in my case, I've escaped more or less unscathed in my relationships with men but have been vulnerable in friendships. I feel lucky to have a circle of wonderful friends who I met in the land of 'before' who have stuck with me, but in the dark times of my adult life, when my mental health was at its worst, I attracted women who on the surface were saints and saviours. With hindsight, the friendships were not as healthy as ones forged during less vulnerable times.

When these strong and controlling characters, love bombed me with care and affection, quickly inveigling themselves into every corner of my life, I felt flattered initially, lucky even, but never able to articulate what made me uneasy. My gut instinct was there but it was weak, and I ignored it, despite feeling controlled. Weren't they always saying how much they loved me and how important I was to them? Interestingly these were the people to turn away as I became stronger, less 'dependent' when I started on my journey of survivor activism – a hard lesson in the importance of listening to instinct.

In his work on Archetypes, Jung beautifully describes the symbolic meaning of 'the old wise man or woman.' He describes it as being an aspect of 'Self' or one's mana personality – a primordial energy that can either assist growth and transform, or destruct and destroy. To Jung, the Self was the centre of the psyche, where light and dark are brought together in a process known as individuation. In its positive form, the old wise woman acts as a guide to lead an individual on the quest for growth, spiritual knowledge, and self-actualization.

However, Jungian psychology is characterised as 'unscientific'. Archetypes are not something that can be proven by scientific methodology. They are, however, the ingredients of fairy stories, fables and legends found throughout the world, passed down through generations. In the case of Sophie's description of the Old Witch, a pure medical model might see her experience as a visual and auditory hallucination – a sign of pathology. However, when I asked Sophie about the Old Witch, she was able to give a perfectly logical explanation of what she meant for her.

Chapter 3

The Butterfly Queen

good night, I love you he says
breathing whisky
yellowed fingers push and press
body hot and tangled my nightdress
rucked and caught
in a padded cage of feather and down
a part of me dies

Sophie Olson

The Butterfly Queen lived in The Kingdom of His with the Big Princess, the Little Princess and the Evil King. The Little Princess loved the Butterfly Queen very much. Whilst the Evil King dressed in fine black clothes, the Butterfly Queen wore white clothes. Like her daughter, she dressed in rags and scraps, but the Little Princess thought she looked quite beautiful in her white rags and tried to be near to her as much as she could. This proved to be difficult. The Butterfly Queen was usually to be found inside the high walls of The Kingdom, but she was busy and moved quickly, fluttering here and there, inside and outside. The Little Princess thought the fluttering around was fun and exciting but she didn't have wings so she soon grew tired of following and found a safe place in the shadows where she could rest.

One day, the Evil King opened the gate in the high wall and left The Kingdom. The Little Princess saw that he took his Ice and Darkness with him and the sun came out in the cottage. The Little Princess came out of the shadows and the sun came out inside her too. She could feel her Body and it didn't feel Useless anymore. Her arms and legs were lighter. She could move quickly and didn't get so tired.

When the Evil King left for The World, the Little Princess discovered she did have wings after all. They had been curled up and hidden because they didn't want the Cold Ice Eyes to see them.

The Little Princess unfurled her tiny white wings and found that she too could flutter and flit. Here and there and up and down. Together, the Little Princess and the Butterfly Queen fluttered. They flew around the garden and watched the flowers grow. They fed the chickens and they collected the eggs. They laughed and played together. The days went by and the Little Princess began to forget the crawling Snakes, and her bruises and bites began to heal. When she went to bed at night, she tucked her little wings away, content with the day and ready to flutter again tomorrow.

But the one thing about Light is that it is always followed by Dark.

One night, when the Little Princess was sleepy in her bed, a huge Shadow fell over the cottage and the Little Princess's wings withered and died. The Shadow grew bigger and bigger and came closer and closer, and riding on its tail sat the Evil King. Again, he laughed and played even though no one from The World was watching, but this time the Little Princess knew it was a clever Trick. *I don't want to be a Frozen Statue again*, she thought to herself, and turned her face to the wall so as not to see the Cold Ice Eyes.

She didn't freeze to Ice but instead felt herself drowning as the huge Shadow covered her Body. She tried to fight it, but she was too Useless and Weak. As the Shadow came over the Little Princess, it started to swallow her up. Firstly, it swallowed her feet, then her legs, Body, arms, hands and mouth, until all that was left of the Little Princess were her eyes and ears.

She remembered she could escape with her eyes, but the window was dark; it was night and the Little Princess couldn't see where to go.

She couldn't hear the birds, as they were fast asleep. She could hear the Butterfly Queen, but she was too busy fluttering here and there. She couldn't hear the Old Witch but knew she was watching. She could hear the Evil King's breathing and it got louder and louder until it was roaring in her ears and giving her a headache.

The Little Princess could feel the Snakes under the Shadow, and knew she would surely die if she did not escape.

The Little Princess couldn't escape. She felt a thousand crawling Snakes wrap around her Body. The writhing Snakes curled around her ankles, and they crawled up her legs.

'I am going to die,' said the Little Princess to herself.

There were Snakes in her hair and Snakes on her chest and they found ways into the very heart of her, and the Little Princess could feel them bite and crush her little Body.

'I want to die,' said the Little Princess.

The Evil King would not have heard as his roaring was too loud, but her Body, on hearing those words, listened, and bit by bit, pieces of the Little Princess began to wither and die and the Little Princess was glad. When The Snakes stopped crawling, the Little Princess lay still, looking at the wall.

'Goodnight,' said the Evil King and he tucked up the half dead little Body so tightly with the Shadow that it became part of the Little Princess forevermore.

Exploring 'The Butterfly Queen'

To: Sophie
From: Pat
So that, Sophie, is what made you shut down. You could not escape out of the window. It sounds like you had near death experience, but without leaving your body. That is what made you ill in every way, physically and mentally, because on those occasions you could not escape out of the window. It seems to me as if you are now beginning to connect with this little girl, and this is excellent. Talk to her and love her. She needs to be loved and parented.

To: Pat
From: Sophie
I don't think I've ever felt so alone tonight, in a house full of people. Thank you so much for reading it. I have taken up your time today and I do really appreciate your help. These are not recovered memories. I just find it easier to articulate them this way. The car, his bed, the basement, on holiday, in the woods. There's so much more. Most I remember and some I need to work on remembering.
It's hard to love her when I can barely look at her because I see his face in mine.

To: Sophie
From: Pat
This must have been exhausting for you. You have done so well. Detaching the little girl for the moment into a story is the best way to process because it reduces the pain. You may not be ready for some time for using the pronoun 'I' or 'me' until you have me with you. Sleeping in the foetal position might be helpful tonight so you don't feel so alone and vulnerable, and maybe find something to cuddle.

To: Pat
From: Sophie
Is it ok to keep sending you the story?

To: Sophie
From: Pat
Yes, it is, Sophie. I was away at dance class and Qigong but am back now.

> When working with my supervisor, I instinctively knew that less was more. If I were to be supervised within the model of keeping traditional therapy boundaries (fifty-minute sessions, the rule of no in-between session contact, for example) it would have acted like a barbed wire around the work. I would undoubtedly have been told that the boundaries I had put in place around time and familiarity needed review. And yet, it was this lack of restrictions that were making a difference.
>
> However, I was acutely aware that it was essential to work safely and to understand my own limitations. I needed to find a way for me, personally, that would allow me to do this work. This 'way' was acupuncture and Qigong, and along with these disciplines came a 'mentor'. I had already studied for two years in Five Element Qigong. I am currently a Medical Qigong Practitioner continuing to train with a Master with over twenty years' experience in this discipline. I receive regular acupuncture treatments from him to maintain a balanced mind and body. This brings stability to my therapeutic approach and assists me to work from a state of 'true self' as opposed to 'ego self'.
>
> Recently I have begun training with two Chinese Masters in Zhineng Qigong. This approach was developed by Dr Pang Ming who drew on Chinese and Western Medicine to bring a scientific approach to physical and psychological healing.
>
> Receiving Sophie's fairy tale was as powerful for me, as her therapist, as it was for her writing it. It is always a wonderful experience watching clients reach that place of understanding that there is life beyond abuse. I don't think Sophie would ever have released her traumatic story if the powerful tools of writing and drawing had not been introduced. Working with her, I began to realise that something more powerful than her story was emerging.

~ Part Two ~

Acknowledgement

Standing on the Precipice

Summer

It was around this point that sharing my story with Pat impacted directly on my state of mind. My mood began to dip. It was like standing at the top of a cliff with a pair of wings, surveying the horizon and the direction I needed to take from my vantage point, but recognising that to move forward, I had to take a giant leap of faith, not knowing if I would fly, or plummet at high speed towards the jagged rocks below. As I wrote my story, I had no choice but to acknowledge it. I read the chapters repeatedly, often late into the night, not wanting to accept it was my story at all. The words were there and whilst that was better than having them sitting inside me, coming to terms with them, and the abuse, was a different matter.

I was getting to the point in my processing of trauma where I needed (and wanted) to go into more detail about the sexual abuse, but shame and fear of equating these details with my own body held me back. For the first time I began to acknowledge how serious the abuse was and that was challenging because my mantra had always been *'it could have been worse'*. I still struggled to say the word *abuse* out loud and the closest I'd got to saying the word *rape* was describing myself as a survivor of 'attempted' rape, back in the peer support groups – deliberate and carefully considered rewording of reality. I needed to try out the words and I needed validation from Pat, deciding at this point to test the waters and gauge how she might respond if I continued with the fairy tale.

> I have trapped myself upstairs today. I think this has been the worst day. I feel like my soul is dying.
>
> Why is today so bad?
>
> I don't know. I can't face seeing anyone at all.

Then spend time just being and let your husband take care of the children.

I want to ask you a question. It's about rape and what your definition of rape is. I don't think I can ask you in a session, but my mind is fixating on this at the moment, so tomorrow if we have our session, you know where I'm at even if I can't speak it.

Yes, that's fine. Do you want your session at the usual time or earlier?

2.30 is fine. Will you be able to reply before? On here?

Do you want me to type the definition to you?

Yes. Your definition, as a person who works with women like me. Your opinion.

My definition of rape is unlawful sexual intercourse or any other sexual penetration of the vagina, anus, or mouth with another person, whether it's using force or not, without that person's consent. It can either be by use of a penis, or digitally, or use of a foreign object. Basically, any unlawful sexual penetration of another person without their consent. Consent is the key word here. In the case of a minor there can be no consent as they are underage.

I hope you don't think that was a strange thing to ask you.
Not at all. It is very necessary that it is clear for you exactly what it means.

But there is, therefore, a scale, isn't there? Or if not legally, there is in terms of the impact on the person.

For each person the impact is different. I have worked with victims of gang rape in war settings, through to young girls who have been sexually assaulted but not raped, and they can struggle with this as much as my clients who survived gang rape. As I always say, it is not what has happened, it is what it has done to you as a person. For a child, generally the effects are worse because it goes unsaid for so many years and the memories become pushed down even further. The younger the child, the more difficult the recovery can be.

Why do I find it so hard to speak the words?
Do other people find it so hard? I'm just stuck.

Because rape is a horrific word and conjures images of severe trauma. Yes, others do find it hard; they don't want to admit it happened. Often there is a sense of guilt too. Having a loss of control over what happens to you is very frightening, so it can become preferable for survivors to think that it must have happened *because* of something they did or didn't do. That on some level they *must* have been to blame. Alternatively, some try to minimise what happened because they don't want to acknowledge what really happened. There are as many reactions to it as there are impacts of this awful act.

OK. Can we do this bit by bit? I practice telling you something and you give me feedback?

Yes, of course. I am going to drive back home in a minute and then I can pick up from there.

OK. I need to start gradually.
Thank you.

I would like you to take this all at a slow pace so that it doesn't overwhelm you. Slow steps like a child walking for the first time.

Later on . . .

I've sent it in an email.

OK, I'm home now and will take a look.

To: Pat
From: Sophie
Subject: Definition
OK.

   The bath-time abuse I think I was probably 4/5/6 years old. [It] fell under the guise of something 'normal' and it was normal to be washed in the bath.

   However, I just knew, somehow, that it wasn't right. There was no threat, it was very calm in the room. I don't think I was even frightened. Not initially. I was sleepy and the water was warm, and I had his attention. I certainly never protested; it didn't even hurt at first. It felt pleasurable to be touched (that's a very difficult thing to admit to you and is the cause of great angst and inner turmoil) but I still knew it wasn't right.

   When it began to feel uncomfortable, I still just stood there. Then, it did hurt. I thought it had been an accident but when I tried to move away, he didn't take his hand away and he didn't stop. And still, I never said stop or I don't like it. I just stood still. Listening to the noise of the TV below, my mother in the kitchen, the birds scrabbling in their nest on the roof above the sloping ceiling and his breathing. He started to breathe really fast, but I taught myself not to look. They were his fingers, of course, to start with, but in my story they are snakes because it's easier to describe them that way because the thought of him doing that to me is so hard to accept. But 'the snakes' diminish him of responsibility which he must now take. At the very least, in my own mind.

   I waited for him to finish. I was freezing cold and then thought I'd done something wrong as he would finish the bedtime routine, but he would be cross. He was heavy handed as he cleaned my teeth, his hand hurt my face as he gripped it and my neck as he forced it back. He brushed my hair too hard and that hurt too. He barely dried me and forced my nightclothes on over my damp body. Afterwards was when it really hurt. I went to bed with my vagina burning more times than I can remember. This was a frequent occurrence. I would apply a cream I found in the bathroom drawer to myself to soothe the pain because the discomfort was keeping me awake and was unbearable. I knew not to tell my mother. I was ashamed to be looking through the drawers for cream and I was as quiet as I could be. I was on high alert, listening out for any sound of footsteps coming up the stairs. His, but mainly hers. I don't remember him telling me to not tell her, but I just knew not to.

The physical soreness confirmed I had done something wrong as it felt like a consequence to something I didn't understand.

It has just occurred to me that this abuse was the precursor to the bedroom abuse when he would come to say goodnight. That bath-time 'washing' probably stopped because I grew too big to be washed in the bath.

This makes sense now that I've pictured myself as about 7-9 when the snakes came to my bed.

I'm really sorry if it's too graphic. Let me know if you need me to tone it down a bit.

I'd really appreciate feedback on this one. Thank you.

To: Sophie
From: Pat
Thank you for this explanation, and it's brilliant that you have taken it to your adult self to explain it for the child. It feels like you and the child 'you' are finally connecting. Let's deal with the angst and inner turmoil part first.

The water was warm and comfortable and pleasurable. To be touched intimately, and for a young child to react, is not abnormal (you can look at this online about early sexualisation of children if you wish). The sexual response is your autonomic nervous system, so there is no control over this response. Many women after rape will be horrified that they have a sexual response sometimes, even orgasm, when they have flashbacks/nightmares. So, remember this part of the body comes under automatic responses. If a child is awakened early, sexually, they may become promiscuous because of it. Also, some young children – I don't know about girls because I have only raised boys – will touch themselves from a very young age once a nappy is taken off. When I say young, I remember being surprised seeing it at younger than twelve months old. Young children will explore these pleasure zones and the area will respond. I hope this clarifies this for you and you can begin to address the turmoil.

The response is normal but the adult creating such a response is NOT. The child may well have a feeling that it is not right as I think children often have a sense that this is a very 'special' part of their body. The age of 4 to 6 would be a good indication that you did not understand what was going on and could not give it words, as you wouldn't have such words. Snakes therefore are a good description. During the bath episode he combined pleasure and pain as all perpetrators do . . . It is typical head-working stuff and leaves a victim totally confused. You may want to go online and find a book called *Living with the Dominator* by Pat Craven. There is also an online course called The Freedom Programme based on the book. Although designed to help victims of domestic abuse, by describing the perpetrator's behaviour it will give you an insight and validation of the type of behaviour a perpetrator uses. The chapter on 'the head worker' is particularly useful, and you can adapt it from the woman to the child in your case.

Do not concern yourself about being too graphic. Also, you are now 'voicing' it in written form and allowing the child to have the language they did not have. This is all so, so, awful but I want you to be really proud of yourself. Well done.

To: Pat
From: Sophie
Well, as you know, I find the body memories the hardest legacy of child abuse.

Even though I have full understanding of why that happens, it doesn't make it easier. My sexual responses became heightened as a child, but all mixed up and sexual response wasn't pleasurable, it was comparable to feeling a wave of nausea, or a headache. Something to dread and fear.

I would be interested to know what my teachers had observed as I think I did touch myself often as a young child, until I learnt acceptable social norms. I remember the shame of being noticed by one teacher when I was 7. From a psychologist's point of view, an abused child may be seen as sexually precocious and may engage in sexual acts, e.g. masturbation, but it's interesting that for me, my memory is so clear about this – when I touched myself, it was not masturbation. I was simply trying to tear away the body memories because they were deeply unpleasant. In the same way a child might grip tightly to a hurt knee or bumped head, I would also touch myself when I was sore and hurting.

These responses are now body memory and I want to be free of them.

Does what happened in this chapter fall under the definition of rape?

OK, the exact crime name for what he did would be 'sexual assault by penetration'. Our laws are different from the US. But the crime I have stated is a serious enough offence to be tried in a Crown Court and for a minor this offence would carry a heavy sentence.

But you knew this already? I've spoken about this before, haven't I?

Yes, you have. I documented it in notes for you, and you had also written about the soreness and the cream and an episode at school where you couldn't sit properly, and a teacher was watching you trying to self soothe.

So sexual assault by penetration isn't actually rape. I'm confused by the definition.

Is it OK to be texting you at this time?
Yes, it's fine. We differentiate in the law to specify exactly what has happened. Of course, it is realistically rape, but the crime would be tried as sexual assault by penetration in a court. I think it's important to put it all together because it seems his 'sexual assaults' got worse as time went on.

My body memories are raising their ugly head again.

Gather them together and tell them very sternly that today is not the day . . . The sun is shining . . . I am alive, and I am going to make the best of these precious moments of my life.

No, it doesn't work like that unfortunately. They have a mind of their own and go when they go.

Flashbacks

I had a very real flashback last night with sound. It was as if I was there.

Do you want to text it to me or send an email, or save it for Friday?

It wasn't much. Nothing new, I was in the bath, and I could feel the warmth of the water and hear the sounds very clearly. The new bit was seeing his hand under the water. It was so real. Like I'd gone back in time.

OK, really, well done. This is a significant change in your way of processing. It seems to me that since you have used the word rape, you are allowing yourself to process this. This was the 'blocking' word. Now that it has been unblocked, I suspect that gradually more will be accessed. I would like you to write it in your book as a new memory and then let it rest. Try not to overwhelm yourself, and allow this new information to slowly sink in. Remember, all this time you were living with a monster and as you know the child could say and do nothing. They were invisible and silent to the outside world.

I can't say that word out loud. It's a hard day today.

Don't worry about not being able to say the word out loud . . . you have written it.

I still don't know if I can trust it.

Don't worry about trusting what you are getting. Just write it down and see what else follows . . .

Chapter 4

All the Wrong Things

'But it's no use now,' thought poor Alice, 'to pretend to be two people! Why, there's hardly enough of me left to make one respectable person!"

– *Alice's Adventures in Wonderland*, Lewis Carroll

'Stand up,' said the Evil King.

The Little Princess stood and watched as the Evil King removed his watch and placed it at the end of the bath, near the taps. She watched as he unbuttoned his cuffs and rolled up his shirt sleeves and she watched his hands as they lathered the soap he took from the rack.

As the Little Princess waited, she watched the shadows as they shimmered and shifted on the surface of the bath water. It made her feel peaceful and sleepy. Then she noticed something was Wrong.

It was Wrong that her legs were warm but only from her knees down to her feet and her body was cold from her head down to her knees. It was Wrong that she was standing for this long. It was Wrong that she was hurting. It was Wrong that she knew it was Wrong but she couldn't say so to the Evil King because he was too busy making all the things Wrong. He was hurting her.

And The Little Princess wondered about The Wrong and continued to stand in the middle of all these Wrong things and tried not to be there at all but then the sounds began to go Wrong too.

The sound that was most Wrong was the Butterfly Queen, fluttering and flitting beneath The Little Princess's feet, under the hard enamel of the bathtub, through the old carpet and dusty floorboards, beneath the kitchen ceiling and in the kitchen itself, directly underneath the Little Princess and the Evil King, who was doing All The Wrong things above her head.

Breathing, thought the Little Princess. The breathing was Wrong. Breathing was in and out and calm and soft. It was bedtime stories, resting her head on her the Butterfly Queen's chest and hearing her heartbeat.

She could hear the Evil King breathe. This breathing was the jagged catch of freshly cut fingernails on a knitted jumper. This was uneven. It was panting, like her dog in the sun. It was in and out – a hiss on the in and a whistle on the out. *Hiss. Whistle. Hiss. Whistle.* The Little Princess couldn't stop her ears from listening. She imagined the air rushing past a million nose hairs like a foul wind blowing through the trees and it made her feel sick.

Stop. She wanted him to stop.

Stop. She wanted to say.

Stop. Breathing.

She couldn't say stop because she was caught in a trap by his hands, by the jagged and uneven sounds and by All The Wrong Things. She handed herself to the Evil King because there was nothing else she could do.

Even Wrong Things come to an end and the Little Princess slipped under the water to warm her shivering little body. She soon found herself being lifted out of the bath and in front of the Evil King who wrapped her in her towel. She felt proud of herself. That had been horrible, thought the Little Princess, but she hadn't Made A Fuss, she had been Good, and she waited for the Evil King's praise.

But the Evil King wasn't happy. The Little Princess felt his Cross as he dried her roughly with the scratchy towel, but only parts of her, leaving the rest wet and cold. Her nightdress stuck to her damp skin and the Evil King tugged and pulled at it in irritation.

'Open your mouth,' he said. 'Hurry up,' he said, and he gripped the Little Princess's chin with one hand and jabbed the toothbrush painfully at the Little Princess's teeth and gums, making her eyes water.

Then, he picked up a hairbrush and began to brush her

hair. Too fast. Too hard and the Little Princess's head jerked backwards.

'When I was a Little Prince', said the Evil King, 'The Matriarch brushed my hair every night for one hundred strokes.'

So the Little Princess braced herself, but the Evil King gave up because he was too Cross and bored of her now, and he took the Little Princess to her bed with her legs still wet and said goodnight with a frown and no story and no tucking in and the Little Princess lay in the dark, feeling cold and sore and wondering what she'd done wrong.

As she lay in the dark, the Little Princess's ears remembered the hiss, whistle and pant.

As she closed her eyes her Body remembered the washing, her mouth remembered the toothbrush and her hair remembered the hairbrush. She didn't like these feelings or these sounds. She didn't like making the Evil King Cross. She didn't like not being Good enough and she began to cry until her pillow was wet with tears. When she awoke the next morning, the Little Princess found her pillow had stuck to her cheek.

In our sessions, Sophie shared a recurring dream she had throughout her childhood. In the dream there was an old house. An old woman lived in this house and Sophie would follow her around as she showed her the different rooms. Sophie never saw her face, only her back. The house was grand, opulent, and beautiful: long corridors filled with antiques; velvet floor-length curtains, and wood-panelled walls. When Sophie and the Old Woman got to the top floor – the attics – the floors were bare boards, and it was dirty and cold. As Sophie followed the Old Woman up the stairs, the stairs started to crack and break, finally collapsing entirely, with both falling to their death. Sophie would wake up at this point.

On reflection, I realised that this dream of the old house was significant in understanding Sophie's fairy story, and the abandonment Sophie felt. Downstairs on the ground floor, everything appeared normal – in fact, the downstairs was beautiful, opulent, and perfect. But upstairs was very different. Upstairs, Sophie's world was falling apart and there was no way for her to get down to The Butterfly Queen, and The Butterfly Queen certainly did not come upstairs to rescue Sophie. The 'staircase' was missing.

Earlier in Sophie's therapy, I referred to the perpetrator as being 'a very sick, dead-eyed person'. Some professionals might suggest that this is a controversial thing to say. It could be argued that perpetrators also have their story to tell, and they may have been victims in life. However, when working with survivors of CSA, I have often found that they are searching for a reason to carry 'the blame, shame and guilt' of their abuser, believing they must have done something to make it happen. It felt important to Sophie's therapy that I expressed to her the true horror of The Evil King's behaviour. That here was a person of narcissistic and psychopathic tendencies. I wanted to give validation to Sophie's experience that this person was indeed a person of monstrous proportions, not just in comparative size to the child that Sophie was, but in form also. For Sophie he exuded a terrifying dark force. Sophie, like many survivors do, describes his eyes as being 'ice cold and piercing'. As if there is no soul behind them. Like many perpetrators of abuse, he was a Dr Jekyll and Mr Hyde character, one that appears to the outside world as all good, but behind this appearance, lay something dark and sinister, and of a shocking nature. This was Sophie's daily reality as a child.

Chapter 5

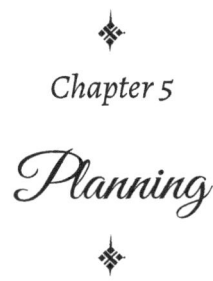

Planning

'Will you hold your tongue!' screamed the cat. 'Another word, and I devour you too!' And the poor little mouse, having 'All-gone' on her tongue, out it came, and the cat leaped upon her and made an end of her. And that is the way of the world.

– Household Stories, the Brothers Grimm

The Evil King had a plan. He had felt her soul leave the Little Princess's Body when he released the Snakes, and he was angry that she had gone. Fear, for him, was the most delicious nectar. When the Snakes were crawling over the Little Princess, delicate wisps of Fear would rise from her skin, and he would enjoy catching them on his Evil tongue. They would quench a great thirst that he felt deep inside his Ugly body.

He was angry because when the Little Princess left her Body, she took her Fear with her, and he had nothing to drink. *How dare she*, thought the Evil King, and he watched her carefully with his Cold Ice Eyes to see how she did it. He soon understood that her Body and mind were separate, and whilst her Body would remain, it was her mind that left, and it was her mind that held the deepest depths of her soul and was where she kept her hope, her courage, and her love. The Evil King wondered if hope, courage, and love tasted as sweet as the beautiful Fear and was determined to capture the Little Princess's mind and find out.

One morning, the Little Princess awoke and found to her surprise she had grown a tail in the night. It was long and pink and scaly. She got out of bed and stood up. The tail reached all the way to the floor and followed the Little Princess wherever she went. She looked in her mirror and saw two furry little ears sticking out of the top of her head and whiskers poking through her little face.

'Oh!' said the Little Princess, but it came out like a squeak. *I am a mouse*, thought the Little Princess curiously.

At breakfast, the Butterfly Queen didn't seem to notice the Little Princess's long tail, she didn't seem to feel the furry ears when she stroked the Little Princess's head, and she didn't seem to hear the squeaks when the Little Princess asked for *more milk, please*. The Little Princess was even more curious. *How strange*, she thought.

The Evil King walked into the room and sat down at the table. In the night, changes had happened to him too. His hands had turned into huge black paws, with sharp black claws. On the top of his head, he had two large black furry ears and behind him a long, black and bushy tail that he flicked backwards and forwards.

The Butterfly Queen didn't seem to notice the changes in the Evil King either and carried on with her fluttering.

The Evil Cat looked at The Little Mouse Princess. He licked his paws and preened his whiskers. A Shadow fell over the cottage and The Little Mouse Princess quivered in her chair. The Evil Cat flexed his claws and looked some more at The Little Mouse Princess, trying to see where she was hiding her mind. The Little Mouse Princess hid her face the best she could behind her hands and ran and hid.

The Butterfly Queen fluttered here and there and didn't seem to notice, and The Evil Cat smiled.

Exploring 'Planning'

Emotional abuse is integral to CSA and in my case, it was part of the manipulation and grooming process necessary to ensure my silence. Abuse and threats to myself and to the people I loved were mirrored in the abuse of animals. Psychological manipulation was constant and left me in a state of heightened anxiety, with the brain and body becoming hypervigilant. I never really left this state of being and even now find it very difficult to relax. I've tried mindfulness, Reiki, Pilates, yoga, meditation, walking, breathing techniques, but true relaxation – genuine, authentic peace – does not come naturally to me. I believe the emotional abuse rewired me. It is one of the many lasting consequences of childhood trauma. I knew that for Pat to truly understand my level of fear and my poor mental health I needed to make the extent of the emotional abuse clear.

> Hi Sophie, I know it's late but I'm picking this up again. You are writing this so well and I hope you are managing to detach from the horror, but this style seems to be working really well for you. Keep going.

I appreciated Pat's response to *Planning* and was encouraged to write the next chapter.

Chapter 6

Mind Capture

When we get to the end of the story, you will know more than you do now ...

– *The Snow Queen*, Hans Christian Andersen

The Evil King was working very hard on hatching a plan to capture the Little Princess's mind once and for all. In the evenings, after his visits to the Little Princess's bedroom, satiated and replete with his feast of delicious nectar, he would shut himself in a dark and dusty shed where he kept a Big Black Book. The Big Black Book was called *How to Capture Minds and Other Projects*. The Evil King would sit himself down on a high stool and lay out the Big Black Book on the workbench. Under the light of the bare bulb above, he studied the book well into the night and, in time, became very knowledgeable.

One morning, when the Little Princess awoke, her head was full of angles, squares and triangles. Their sharp corners poked and scraped, and the Little Princess cried and cried.

The Evil King was nearby.

'What's wrong?' he asked, and he sounded so kind and gentle that the Little Princess forgot for a moment that he was an Evil King and told him about the terrible pain inside her head.

He pulled her close and whispered kindly and gently into her ear. 'You have a headache. I will take away your pain.'

And the Little Princess, in her desperation to be free of the terrible, tortuous agony, trusted the Evil King.

The Evil King placed his large hands on either side of the Little Princess's little blonde head and began to press. With relief, the Little Princess felt the pain recede and was grateful to the Evil King, but then, when her pain had nearly disappeared completely, a terrifying thing happened.

A Shadow fell over the cottage and the Little Princess was suddenly terribly afraid.

She tried to move her head away from the giant hands, but the Evil King pressed harder.

The Butterfly Queen didn't seem to notice the Shadow and she didn't seem to notice that the room had turned Icy Cold.

The more the Little Princess pulled away, the harder the Evil King pressed, until the Little Princess feared that her skull would surely implode into a million pieces.

She opened her mouth to cry out for help, but as she started to speak, the Evil King pressed so hard that the Little Princess felt her skull begin to crack and the Butterfly Queen didn't notice.

I will die now, thought the Little Princess, and the Evil King, hearing her mind, smiled.

Just as she thought she could live not one second longer, the Evil King released his powerful grip and,

Click, click, whirr, click.

The Little Princess saw that the angles and squares and triangles inside her head were, in fact, cameras. Cameras that the Evil King had somehow placed inside her mind. They photographed the Evil King's hands, they photographed his Evil smile, they photographed the Little Princess's limp Body and her tear-stained face. They photographed the Butterfly Queen fluttering, and the photographs in her mind stacked themselves into piles and arranged themselves neatly in a box labelled, *Skull- Crushing Day*.

The Little Princess ran into her safe place and tried to shake out the box of photographs. It refused to fall out of her mind, so she tried to destroy it instead. She hit her head hard with her hands and even harder against the wall, but the box of photographs was stuck fast.

The Little Princess lay down and curled up small and held her teddy close to her face. Now she understood. It had all been a clever Trick and her Useless self had fallen for it.

She knew the box of photographs and the cameras would remain inside her mind forever more and she would never forget and never be free.

Exploring 'Mind Capture'

Flashbacks are a vital part of a survivor's story. These are pieces of the trauma puzzle that, bit by bit, can be pieced together to create a picture of what they have experienced. For many survivors of CSA, they become stuck at the emotional age the child was when they first experienced the abuse. Simple tasks might cause a survivor such intense anxiety that it leads to a panic attack. Some approach adult life with a child's emotional response. Flashbacks are particularly terrifying because they carry fragments of unprocessed physical, emotional, and mental pain. By suppressing them or medicating them, they lie dormant and are never processed. Often, it is only a matter of time before they will re-emerge, sometimes requiring higher doses of medication to keep them under control. Ultimately this results in feelings of numbness and an inability to access emotions.

In Sophie's story she 'takes photos' of each event and stores them. It was her daughter's ninth birthday celebration, the age Sophie was when Sophie's abuse was at its peak, that triggered her inability to cope with them anymore. When flashbacks build to a crescendo, they are like the darkest hours before the dawn – and this is the time when a client is most likely to pose a high suicidal risk. Psychological trauma experienced in childhood requires no different an approach than someone with an acute physical trauma. Patients with acute physical trauma would be admitted to an intensive care unit and given around the clock treatment by a dedicated team. Imagine this patient being told by their team that they were now going off duty and would be returning after one week, and in the meantime the patient would need to care for themselves? It wouldn't happen, but it is how we currently treat survivors of abuse. We need to build intensive care teams for psychological trauma, so that when the flashbacks and panic attacks occur, usually in the middle of the night, a trained member of staff is there to process this with the patient or client in a warm, caring environment, with a hand to hold if necessary and a space to allow them to tell their terrifying story of a child who was abandoned and silenced by physical and psychological terror.

Just on the train to London so picking up emails again . . . Do you know what the black book and him having that shed was all about? I cannot believe that such an evil brutal person has not destroyed many others. Maybe they are too far into psychosis to be able to function. Keep sending me everything that is flowing for you.

It was a Reader's Digest book. I don't know why I wrote about it like that.
None of this was out in the open. I think we all suffered but on our own. It wasn't really discussed.
When he did that to my head, it was in front of [others] but they didn't notice, and I stayed silent. But I thought I was going to die.

[They] didn't notice anything at all did they . . . not the fear in your eyes nor the brutality of this monster. There are so many times where you could have died.

Or maybe I just felt I could have died. He was perfectly in control of the situation. Just because it's how it made me feel doesn't mean it was real, if you see what I mean. He played these mind games.
It's so hard to explain.

I understand what you mean. But whether it was 'real' or not, the fear he instilled in you made it real. One can die of fear and what he did was particularly dangerous for a young child and at such an age when they could make no sense of what was happening. It reminds me of birds in a cage, waiting to be killed . . . They are taken out, one at a time and the other birds know something fearful is happening, but they do not know what. They do know that the other birds never return, and their fear rises, until they almost kill themselves in the cage in a desperate attempt to survive. I have seen this happen in an outdoor restaurant in India where customers choose their meal.

It's hard today. I feel like I've put one foot back in the past and it's hard to stay fully present. Time is passing either too fast or too slow. I have an urge to be totally by myself, but I can't because it's half term.

So maybe time to have a break and have some fun and joy with the children. Pick up again later. You will not lose anything that you have started because the mind is keen to continue whatever it can.

Chapter 7

The Escalator and the Red Boots

Never had she danced so beautifully; the sharp knives cut her feet, but she did not feel it, for the pain in her heart was far greater.

– The Little Mermaid, Hans Christian Andersen

One day the Little Princess, the Big Princess, the Butterfly Queen and the Evil King were in The World.

They were shopping in a huge shop and the Little Princess was fascinated by the moving staircases.

'They are called escalators,' said the Evil King.

'Be careful,' said the Butterfly Queen, 'hold on to the Evil King's hand.'

The Evil King looked at the small blonde princess hopping with excitement in her little red rubber boots and an idea popped into his head. It was too good an opportunity to miss, he thought. He was, after all, feeling a bit thirsty and could do with some delicious nectar.

He waited until the Butterfly Queen had fluttered off somewhere else, then he knelt and looked at the Little Princess with his Cold Ice Eyes. The Little Princess wasn't unduly worried by this, as they were in The World and she'd never been turned into a Frozen Statue in The World before.

'Escalators are fun,' said the Evil King gently, 'but they can be dangerous. You must never go on by yourself. Always hold my hand and don't let go, whatever you do.'

The Little Princess nodded. She understood and she so wanted to ride up and down. 'I will count to three and then, together, we will step on. What must you not do?' asked the Evil King.

'Let go of your hand,' replied the Little Princess.

'Good girl,' said the Evil King, standing up again and the Little Princess felt proud.

Hand in hand, the Little Princess and the Evil King walked to the top of the escalator. It was shiny and fast, and it whirred and rolled.

'Ready?' said the Evil King.

'Ready!' said the Little Princess.

He started to count, slowly and clearly. 'One, two, three –'

And the Little Princess stepped onto the top shiny disappearing step, and the Evil King did not. He stood still, gripping the Little Princess's hand. Only then, with a flash of pain in her heart, did the Little Princess realise she had been Tricked.

She was suspended, hanging by one small arm and cried out in fear to the Evil King, but he didn't pull her back up, and he didn't step on, he looked at her, with his Cold Ice Eyes and smiled a slow smile. Her arm felt like it was being ripped from her little Body as the shiny, rolling machine did its best to carry her down and the Evil King did his best to keep her suspended.

She tried to pull herself up and scramble up the sharp-edged metal stairs, but they were too fast, and the jaws of the escalator opened and clamped down on her little red boot.

She cried out in pain to the Evil King, as she felt the metal teeth rip through the rubber boot and press onto her small leg but the Evil King just looked and watched and smiled and licked his lips and the delicious nectar rose in wispy tendrils from the Little Princess's skin.

When she accepted she would be swallowed up forever and stopped fighting it, she saw, through her tears, the frantic fluttering of the Butterfly Queen who appeared behind the Evil King, and the look of horror on her face.

Only then did the Evil King pull up the Little Princess by her arm in one quick movement, and with cries of alarm and words of comfort, he gathered her into his arms and cradled her and wiped the tears from her face and the blood from her leg.

The Little Princess flopped in his arms and watched. She watched the people of The World and wondered and wondered how they had not seen. She watched the Butterfly Queen fluttering and stroking and dabbing and worrying and trying to fix her little broken daughter. And she watched the Evil King and he saw her looking. And as he locked his Cold Ice Eyes onto hers and smiled, she heard him whisper in his rotting heart, *I can make you dead, if I choose to,* and the Little Princess understood completely and stayed silent.

The cameras clicked and whirred, and the photographs stacked themselves neatly into a box labelled, *Escalator Day.*

Exploring 'The Escalator'

I remember this escalator episode [from our sessions]. Also, strange that no one else saw what was going on enough to intervene. Maybe it all happened so fast? He must have chosen his moment. How old were you here?

It happened very fast and didn't last for long. Seconds rather than minutes. However, I knew it was deliberate. It is one of my clearest memories and I'll never forget him just holding me and his smile and making no attempt to pull me back up. I also know it wasn't accidental although he made it look like an accident.
I don't know about other people. Maybe he just chose his moment or maybe there weren't many people there at that moment.
My age? This I'm unclear about. Older than 3, younger than 7.

Autumn

Around this time of therapy with Pat I watched a documentary about 'Genie', a child victim of severe abuse. I had first heard her story during an A Level psychology lesson about language acquisition, triggering a flashback to a time in childhood where I was 'tricked' into taking part in a cruel game. My memory of this event was very clear, but I had no memory of the time immediately before or after this 'game'. It was a carefully preserved moment in time and a memory I'd shelved for many years, and never forgotten. Watching the documentary reminded me both of how I'd felt during the lesson and as a child. I experienced old and familiar feelings of detachment that in the past hadn't ended well – usually resulting in self-injury or suicidal ideation.

Instead of self-harming I wrote *The Cage* and sent it to Pat. I voiced these feelings of detachment in the messages because it felt safer to be written out and discussed than to be kept inside.

> **Would you say it's normal to feel detached after our session as the days have gone on? I'm feeling safe but absent and feel like I'm losing periods of time. I hope you don't mind me messaging.**

> No, it's absolutely fine to message and yes, detachment and dissociation is a very common coping mechanism. It is less destructive, because ultimately a detachment from this awful stuff is what you are looking for. Eventually you can attach to the present instead and take your life forward.

> **That's helpful to know. Because I did it so much as a child, I assumed it was a negative thing.**

> No, it is a protective thing, particularly going out of body as a child. I will explain that a little more when we meet.

> **I've just watched a short documentary on the case study of Genie. I remember what I identified with and still do. It triggered feelings of isolation and loneliness that she would**

have felt, being cut off from the world by an abuser who had the control.

OK that's good you have identified with what it was. Allow yourself to breathe those emotions out and don't get overwhelmed by them. We will look at these together and I will also re-look at this story and get an insight into it myself.

OK, but it's very important that I'm not giving you the wrong impression and that you think my experiences were worse than they were. What happened to Genie was a whole different level of child abuse and not comparable.

It's never about the level of abuse experienced, it is about what it does to the individual person.

Looking at what it does is a challenge, I think because I've always told myself that it wasn't that bad.

And normalising awful things is a coping mechanism.

Chapter 8

The Cage

Before the castle gate all was as the fox had said: so the son went in and found the chamber where the golden bird hung in a wooden cage.

— *The Golden Bird*, The Brothers Grimm

The Little Princess was playing in the garden and the Evil King was digging the vegetable patch. The air was warm, and the sun was bright.

The chickens scrabbled and squabbled for worms as the fresh soil was turned over by the steely edge of the sharp spade.

With a flapping commotion of feather and dust, a brown hen shot out of the henhouse, shouting her frantic announcement to The Kingdom of His. The Little Princess went to look. She loved to be the first to discover the delight of a freshly laid, warm, speckled egg and would scoop it up and carry it proudly before her in two hands, carefully, slowly, one foot in front of the other and take it to the kitchen, where the Butterfly Queen would put it in a bowl with the others.

The Little Princess skipped back outside and carried on with the games in her head. She imagined she was riding a pony. She jumped over the daffodils and galloped up and down the lawn. She reared and bucked and kicked and whinnied and the Evil King, stopping to rest, leaned on his spade and watched.

He called to the Little Princess and she trotted and jumped across the grass and around the flower beds and onto the raw, earthy patch where the Evil King stood.

'Phew,' said the Evil King, mopping his brow. 'Hot today. Time for a break?' and he asked the Little Princess if she'd like to listen to a story.

The Little Princess was pleased. She wanted his love because she loved him and eagerly lapped up anything that he threw her way. She reminded herself that she mustn't look at his eyes, just in case, but the sun was warm and the flowers were growing and the chickens were slit-eyed and content as they basked in the dusty soil, clucking gently nearby.

The Evil King found a chair to sit in and he pulled the Little Princess close.

'My story', he said, 'is about a little girl.'

'Like me?' asked the Little Princess.

'Yes,' said the Evil King. 'She was a little girl, just like you, and she lived with a Mummy and a Daddy, but one day, her Mummy and her Daddy decided they didn't want a little girl anymore.'

The Little Princess thought about this. She felt worried.

'So what did she do?' asked the Little Princess. She couldn't imagine not having a Mummy and a Daddy anymore.

'Well, she needed someone to look after her, so her mummy and daddy put her in the henhouse and gave her to the chickens to look after instead.'

'I like chickens,' said the Little Princess in a small voice. But her chest felt tight. *How could chickens look after a little girl?* she wondered. *They don't have hands to cook food and they can't speak words, only clucks and squawks.*

'So did the little girl,' said the Evil King. 'At first, she was happy in the henhouse. The chickens were kind to her although she didn't like the chicken food that much.'

The Little Princess thought of the plastic bucket where the Butterfly Queen put the left-over scraps of food that they fed to the hens. Slimy lettuce and mouldy crusts of bread. The Little Princess didn't like her crusts. Or lettuce.

'What happened next?' asked the Little Princess.

'Ah, well, that was the problem,' said the Evil King. 'Little girls grow up. They grow up big and tall. Much bigger than chickens. So one day, when she tried to stand up, she couldn't. The henhouse was too small and the little girl was too big.'

'So what did she do?' asked the Little Princess.

'Well, she had to crouch and that was OK for a while, but she kept growing and growing, so she had to bend over as well until she spent all day and all night curled into a ball.'

The Little Princess was quiet. Her heart fluttered in her chest.

'Did she try to get out?' she whispered.

'She did try, yes. She called out to people nearby to help but it was too late,' said the Evil King.

'Why was it too late?' the Little Princess asked.

'Because by the time she had grown too big to fit in the cage, she had forgotten how to speak human language and could only speak chicken language. When she called for help, all the people heard were clucks and squawks, so no one came to her rescue.'

The Little Princess tried to get down from the Evil King's lap, but he pulled her even closer. She shut her eyes. 'In the end,' he continued, 'someone did notice, and she was rescued, but she never learned how to stand upright again, and she could only speak like a chicken. She flapped her arms and pecked at her food and squawked and clucked forever more.

'The end,' he said.

He pushed the Little Princess off his lap and asked if she had collected the eggs today.

The Little Princess nodded.

'Have you looked in the other hutch?' he asked, and taking her hand, together they walked to the little hutch they sometimes used for the chicks. It was built with a wooden frame and had a triangular roof and came up to the Little Princess's chest. The Evil King unbolted and lifted a small wooden hatch. 'Are there any eggs?' he asked.

'I can't see,' said the Little Princess, peering inside.

'Why don't you get inside and look?' said the Evil King.

The Little Princess knew. Another Trick. Of course.

Stupid, said the Old Witch, from inside her heart.

The sun went in and the air felt cold.

'I don't want to,' she whispered.

The Evil King was firmer. 'Come on,' he said. 'Why don't you pretend you're the little girl in the story? It will be fun. Just pretend.' He looked at the Little Princess and she looked at him and she saw his Cold Ice Eyes and felt herself turning into a Frozen Statue.

'Climb in,' he said, louder this time, and the Little Princess didn't say no because she didn't know how and she did as she was told, as she always had.

She got down on her hands and knees and put her head through the hatch. She could smell the chicken shit and straw and it made her throat itch.

'Come on,' snapped the Evil King impatiently, 'play the game.'

And so the Little Princess crawled into the small cage. She had to curl up small in order to fit her little Body inside and the straw poked her bare legs and hands.

With a loud Bang, the Evil King slammed down the hatch and the Little Princess heard the bolt as he slid it across.

The Little Princess didn't do anything. She didn't shout, she didn't cry, she did nothing at all, she just sat in her cage and put her fingers through the wire and held on tight and watched the Evil King's broad back as he walked away, away, away, towards her house, where the Butterfly Queen was busy fluttering in the kitchen. She breathed and she breathed, and she breathed.

Exploring 'The Cage'

To: Sophie
From: Pat
How did you get out, Sophie? What a terrifying thing to do to a child. This monster has absolutely no redeeming qualities at all, does he? The awful thing was that you knew exactly what was coming but couldn't do a single thing about it.

Looking at this abuse through the eyes of someone else was truly shocking as I saw for the first time how sadistic his behaviour really was.

We Are Not Nervous Patients

At this point in my journey with Pat, my body began to react. I live with chronic pain resulting from conditions I attribute directly to trauma. I was born normally but at the age of eleven developed scoliosis: a degenerative condition of the spine. Because of the abuse that happened to me, I am unable to have the surgery that I've been told could be lifesaving. I have tried having consultations on a few occasions but am too triggered and retraumatised by the medical process and on some occasions by the surgeons themselves. The worst by far was a highly eminent male consultant at a leading orthopaedic hospital, who wagged his finger at me across the desk, saying he would 'section me' if I became distressed and tried to leave my bed during the recovery process. I had given him no reason to suggest I would try to leave but as fear of the consultation made me unable to communicate, I had turned up with a mental health nurse acting as my advocate. This consultants' views around 'mental health patients' was painfully clear to see.

> **I am struggling a lot with my pain levels, yesterday and today. They haven't been this bad for a while now.**
>
> Can you tell me about the pain?
>
> **The pain is through my torso. It affects the point where the worst curvature is but, equally, my lower spine. My ribs are very tight and so is my pelvis. When the pain is very bad, it radiates down my legs. It is worse when the weather is cold and especially damp. I don't get pain in my neck. Standing is an effort and sitting, unless I can sit on a sofa with my legs under me, and breathing is painful and tight. It feels like being in a vice or squeezed in a hug too hard. Lying flat or on heat helps it but when it's like that, the moment I'm upright again, it comes back. A good night's sleep seems to 'reset' it**

and I start again. **It feels like a timer, from the start of the day, working towards the pain.**

Apart from your back, what are you really frightened about at the moment?

I'm not frightened. I'm determined, but it doesn't warrant this pain.

What I would ask you to do over the weekend is to take the chapter 'The Cage' and where possible begin to write this part of the story as 'your' story. The little princess is now Sophie. If it gets too much, leave it and we will see what is there on Monday. Regarding your back, the next thing you may want to consider is what you want to do about your back in the future if the pain is increasing. If you can, go to bed early tonight and text me when you are lying down. Have you got some help with the children?

My husband is helping. He put them to bed while I lay flat on my back.

Good, that's good he is helping. Let me know how you feel writing this, Sophie. I will pick up in a little while.

**I feel detached. Sorry.
Maybe it will be better if I speak it and use 'I' rather than 'she.'**

Yes, that's fine. I just wanted you to make some inroads on this chapter.

It's a start I suppose.

My condition is idiopathic – in other words, there is no known cause.
When I was diagnosed, even at that young age I knew the cause, I was sure of that. It was sexual abuse. It was trauma and it was my subsequent silence.
Abuse was a burden too heavy to carry and this was the

consequence, but I believed it was my fault for not being strong enough to stop my own body from behaving so outrageously. Now I'm in my forties and have to contend with pain, from the severe scoliosis that compromises my heart and lung, and from arthritis in my lower spine. I also have osteopenia in my spine and pelvis. Managing pain is a daily challenge and it is exacerbated by stress, and at this point in therapy, by the release of trauma. It is now acknowledged by some that 'the body keeps the score' – a term coined by Bessel van der Kolk (*The Body Keeps the Score: Mind, Brain and Body in the Transformation of Trauma*).

As an activist, I advocate for accessible healthcare for survivors of CSA. Many survivors find accessing healthcare almost impossible and I look forward to the day in which survivors' needs are recognised. We can be perceived as 'nervous' patients, but this is not the case. We are traumatised by our experiences of abuse and going to the doctor/dentist/nurse/consultant can be triggering and re-traumatising, leaving many of us avoidant. The fault does not lie with us for not being able to 'overcome our fear', it lies with a system that doesn't (yet) understand and accommodate our needs.

A part of my work I'm particularly proud of is The Skylark Project – conceptualised by a collaboration between myself and Dr Charlotte Small, co-lead of the Herefordshire Pain Management Service and clinical lead of the Wye Valley Trust Preoperative Assessment Service. The aims of The Skylark Project are to improve survivor access to healthcare in addition to optimising the quality and experience of the hospital care they receive. I advocate for accessible care because, without it, survivors of CSA will continue to be disadvantaged and they will continue to die. My avoidant nature may be considered extreme by some but how many survivors avoid cervical screening? Prostate checks? How many ignore the lump in their breast because the alternative option of getting help from a system with little understanding of trauma is too frightening to even contemplate?

People present with all sorts of needs. Deaf people require a hearing loop. A wheelchair user will need a ramp to access medical care. A child has different needs to an adult. Someone with dementia has different needs to someone with learning difficulties. This is no different. Survivors have needs that should be accommodated and it is wrong that these are only catered for under the umbrella of 'mental health' because whilst sometimes there will be a crossover, it is not automatic. Identifying these normal responses to trauma as mental health needs risks misunderstanding, unnecessary labelling and survivors feeling disempowered. Survivors' needs resulting from abuse and rape don't automatically equate to 'illness' or 'disorder' and yet that is how they're usually perceived, and this is what needs to change.

~ Part Three ~

Believing, and the Struggles It Brings

Entering the Innermost Cave

Winter

Pat suggested I write *The Cage* as 'my story' and so this is what I did. I went back over it, changing the Little Princess to 'Sophie' and I used the name of the perpetrator instead of the Evil King.

I remember feeling detached as I did this, but it was an important first step into owning my story and paved the way to reading the words aloud when we met face to face during a therapy session, and ultimately to processing this traumatic memory.

I now had a collection of chapters, and they were the most important thing I'd ever created. I began to wonder if they could lend themselves to a book to help others, and as soon as I had this thought, the name of this book came into my head. I mentioned my idea to Pat and told her I would call it *The Flying Child*.

For the first time, despite my survival mechanisms taking control of the feelings emerging, I sensed a glimmer of hope, but going forwards was not straightforward. I was at a crossroads again. I wanted to go in the direction of hope but the pull towards despair and fear was equally strong. I was so tired of fighting to live, and I began to speak openly to Pat about the darkness that enveloped me, and everything I did to keep it at bay. Bulimia was a way of releasing the weight of fear that sat in my stomach and made me feel in control of my weight at a time I was beginning to feel frighteningly out of control. Self-harm was by now regular and hugely risky but it was all I knew. I had no idea how to sit with uncomfortable feelings without resorting to default survival strategies I'd relied upon since childhood. I had never learned how to resolve inner conflict, how to self-regulate without harming or medication, or how to keep myself safe. I was toying with life and death again, but this time under the watchful and distant light of hope.

For the first time ever, birds are appearing in my garden. We have cats and the birds have never really come before even though I encouraged them with feeders. There aren't any feeders anymore but over the last few days, more and more little birds keep appearing. Isn't that amazing?!

Truly amazing and clearly meant for you at this special time.

I failed again, in the end last night.

As Edison said, there is no failure . . . every step is just one step closer to success. Eventually he produced.

I doubt he stuck his fingers down his throat. Wet fingers and electricity would have had a whole different outcome.

Who knows what Edison did . . . he must have been a very angry, frustrated guy at times!

I have cut myself badly tonight.

Why?
So, these are old patterns of behaviour, and are the way an adolescent or a young person in their early twenties might behave. When you are calm, I want you to examine whether this behaviour is appropriate for the adult you are now. If not, then decide which new coping mechanism you want to replace it with. You may want to consider that if you continue to cope in this way, then the very place you don't want to go to may become your only option because you may cut too deeply or your wounds risk becoming infected.

In the moment, it is the safest thing to do because if I don't, I'm frightened that I'll commit suicide, because, in that moment of time, I want to escape. It is a more controlled way of managing that feeling, albeit risky. Followed afterwards by calm, followed by regret and sadness.

OK, so the next big question is, why should you want to be the one to commit suicide? He can never take your mind. That is his big mistake – he hopes and believes his secrets are all his own, because he believes he is invincible but he is not. You have important work to do, Sophie . . . There is no time for checking out.

I don't want to check out but when I get to that point of panic, I self-harm to stop myself from doing worse. It jolts me back to the present. When you say what you said about an adolescent or someone in their twenties behaving like that and if it's appropriate for me now, that makes me feel wretched and ashamed. I don't open up about self-harm because I feel ashamed about it and it's been a big secret. I think that there is a stigma associated with it in older people. I know that it's something that afflicts many people, particularly survivors of abuse. I met people in hospital who are older, yet harming, very secretive about it and deeply ashamed, as I am as it is considered an 'adolescent' behaviour trait. I can see where you're coming from, but it is ingrained in me and I would love help for this. Being honest and letting you know what is going on is such a big step for me and it's because I trust you. Please don't tell me that this behaviour is infantile and inappropriate at the age I am now. I am very, very much aware of that myself, hence the secrecy, and being reminded of that makes me feel like closing up. I am sorry for being blunt. I need to say this as I feel misunderstood. I'm sorry.

I'm glad you are angry about what I have said. I understand why you have the need to do it and that is why I want you to challenge your way of dealing with anger and frustration. I want you to find a healthier way. I want you to consider how you would deal with a family member doing the same thing. What would you suggest to them, as you are very good at managing their behaviour. This behaviour comes from the deeply misunderstood and very frightened child in you; a child that can't be heard in any other way. So don't be sorry, instead, what she needs to do is have a good angry shout and she may have to find somewhere safe to do this.

I think that the emotion I feel about what you said isn't anger, it's fear that you won't understand. Self-harm is the result of anger and panic, yes.

OK, so fear is a good one . . . Get to the other side of it and you have conquered it. If something someone says makes you react deeply, then ask why. If it isn't touching a nerve, then let it go, but if it is, keep challenging yourself . . . Do you need to feel the fear that I won't understand, and if I don't understand, then how can you explain it to me . . . Give it all a language . . . 'If you don't understand me then . . .' what? Add the words.

Fear, because if I feel misunderstood with this, then I begin to lose trust, and without trust then we can't carry on the good work that we were doing. I was made to feel ashamed for being mentally unwell, so I learned to not say anything to anyone. My behaviours – my drinking, self-harm, bulimia – became so secret that I was almost two people. Living two lives. Nobody really knows me at all. I need you to know me so that I can get better.

OK, so that helps me . . . These two people are having a fight with each other . . . One strong and determined, and the other saying, 'I just can't do this,' – partly from feeling overcome with it all and partly the fear of what happens if I do overcome it. In a way, the only way to overcome this is to take the trembling child Sophie, give her a big hug and say, I understand you but please don't harm you because you have a very important job ahead of you and you must now get up and do it. It's like raising your own children. On the one hand you give them love and encouragement and on the other you must also give them firm guidance and boundaries. This is what is needed now with Sophie child. She needs to find another way of coping because harming and running away can no longer be her coping mechanism if she wants to make a difference in this world. You must both love her and guide her firmly.

I can't do that because I hate and loathe her.

So, this is where we need to go in and rescue her. Go back to the photos of the young Sophie . . . The youngest Sophie you can find . . . Possibly the sweet one of her on the lawn where you think abuse might have been beginning to happen but not to the extent it got to by age 9. Take the photo out, put her by your bed. Look at this sweet pretty child and then see if you really want to hate her. Ask yourself why you would want to hate this sweet little child. Keep her by your bed and tell her you are now going to look after her. You may need to draw using your non-dominant hand – work with her so she can draw you pictures and tell you how she feels. She may want to talk to you in a child's voice. Listen to her. She really needs you after all these lonely years.

I can't. I don't want to see my abuser, so I can't look at myself. I'm sorry. I appreciate everything you're saying and I'm sorry that I'm putting barriers up. I'm being totally honest.

That's what I want – honesty. She is not him. There is nothing monster-like about you as I have come to know you. So, imagine you are mirroring him, but you are blinding him with your light and seeking out every bit of his darkness. Change your old perceptions of how you are seeing things and do a mental exercise programme; develop flexibility in your mind. Imagine you are in a mind-gym workout, stretching and bending and twisting until the mind becomes more flexible.

Chapter 9

Mind Capture
(Part 2)

'Since I must die,' answered she (looking upon him with her eyes all bathed in tears), 'give me some little time to say my prayers.'
'I give you,' replied Blue Beard, 'half a quarter of an hour, but not one moment more.'

— *Blue Beard*, Charles Perrault

The Little Princess felt different. She had been born, as all babies are, with love and loyalty in her heart and whilst she loved the Evil King still, the more he captured her mind, the harder her heart became.

The Evil King was ready for Part Two of the plan.

His visits to the Little Princess's bedroom continued but always under the cover of darkness. That was the only way to ensure that her mind didn't escape into the sky.

The Evil King was becoming bored and frustrated by this. He was thirsty in the daytime and on his trips to The World and he wanted access to the Little Princess's delicious Fear whenever he desired. It was his right, after all.

He had noticed the Little Princess worried that she may die at his hands but now he needed her to be sure and convinced that he could easily end her life if he so wished. This knowledge would shackle more of her mind, thus making it harder for her to escape out of the window.

I Don't See Much Point to This Anymore

I've gone down again very quickly and don't see much point to this anymore. I want my children to be able to live a more normal life than they do with me.

> I think it's time to tell your husband what is going on for you because it's not fair to him or the children.

**Yes. You're right. I'm not strong enough for this.
He doesn't want to hear it. He's heard it before. It's no one's job to fix me, so little point in hearing it.
I am in so much pain. It hurts to breathe and to stand and to even lie down and sleep. I am never pain free and I'm so tired of it. My ribs and my spine hurt as well as my neck, even down through my hips, legs, and knees. I'm tired. Really, really tired. I don't know how to manage the housework, cooking and working. I can barely stand.**

> You need to rest and then have a chat tomorrow about how this might be managed.

My husband has said that he thinks I need to go to the hospital.

> What do you think?

I don't feel very safe.

> Then you should listen to that voice. If you don't feel safe, then you need to go somewhere you can feel safe. If your husband is saying the same thing, then it's time to listen. You haven't felt safe for some days and that is why I suggested you tell him so that he understands what is going on.
> Are you able to do a call with [psychiatrist] and then she can

assess from her point of view whether it's better to take you in or not?

I just need to be stronger. I have taken slow-release tramadol today. Maybe that will help. I need to manage my pain.

Yes, if you are in pain that doesn't help, but do the phone call as well.

I think I'll wait. She knows me so well and has seen me at my worst and when normal. She doesn't take admissions lightly as she knows how phobic I am. I know she will think I should be admitted, and I'm frightened to be honest with her in case the control is taken away from me.

So, you have the choice of either going to hospital or staying at home and managing it. I would strongly suggest you get your husband on board so that he knows what is happening and can monitor the safety situation from everyone's point of view.

He is fully aware.
What must you think of me?

As I have always said, I think you are an amazing person. I understand very well how much easier it is to return to being a victim, than struggling to be a survivor. The resilient mind gets worn down under pressure . . . but if you survived everything that you have . . . There must be a reason and I think you know what that is. If someone has had to endure so much abuse, then all one can do with that is to go out there and make a difference, and that, lovely Sophie, is your greatest fear. Going out there . . . making a difference and changing your life as you change others.

I think you're right but sometimes I don't think it's as simple as having the right mindset. Over the last few days, I don't feel as if I have a choice and my brain is letting me down. I don't feel AT ALL comfortable being in 'victim' mode and every day I wake up feeling positive and then it starts to slip away from me.

Without getting too bogged down in it . . . think of it like this. Your mind spent years being conditioned by the abuse you endured. You had so much to deal with. Now think about the difficulty in trying to change that conditioning quickly without the programme in place to do it. You have had years of punishing conditioning and no one to teach you even the most basic lessons in survival, let alone how to find a way out and really thrive! So, it's scary . . . like being on an open road with no driving skills and traffic coming from every direction. You are right, it's not just the right mindset, it's the reigning of that mind, every day, like a physical workout until it knows only how to thrive.

What do you advise about pain? I'm in so much pain. I've taken 100mg tramadol and it's barely touched the sides. I can sort of feel like I've taken it but not really. It's not a tolerance thing because I haven't taken it for a few months. I save it for emergencies. It used to do something but now it isn't.

Ease off whatever you are doing that is causing this. Check the tension levels in your body and pinpoint exactly where they are. Massage that area and apply some heat to relax it such as a hot water bottle, and you may need to ask the GP for a different medication.

When it's like this and it hurts to take each breath, I think that if it was my dog, I would have put her to sleep. They've tried diclofenac, patches . . . codeine. I don't want to be a zombie on morphine for the rest of my life. Gabapentin. Pregabalin. Duloxetine. Some side effects are as bad as the pain. They didn't work either.

Is there anything new they could prescribe, such as a muscle relaxant rather than pain relief? Yes some side effects are horrible and morphine is not ideal as it's highly addictive. Have you tried CBD?

I vape it and have tried drops.

Clearly not working either?

No. Thank you. It helps to talk about it. No one really knows how bad my pain can get. I don't really talk about it. My family got used to me saying my back hurts, but I don't think anyone can ever really understand what it feels like unless they've experienced it.
Alcohol is the only thing that helps but my mental health then deteriorates. And my liver most likely. Especially drinking heavily on the top of tramadol.
Massage used to help a lot but it's too triggering to lie on my front and the memories of abuse are too much.

OK, all I can suggest is get back to GP and see what they can do in the way of muscle relaxants as massage clearly worked, so that would suggest that it is the muscles that are completely tensed up.

I can't talk to or see my GP because of my phobia.

Do you not already have a prescription for the meds you take so can't you ask them to change it?

I don't take pain medication regularly anymore. Because at first it works, then it doesn't, but by then I'm very cautious about addiction.

OK, so I would recommend a phone call to [your psychiatrist] anyway. Tell her you would like to manage things if you can, but the pain is getting you down and see what she says.

I know what she'll say.

Later that night.

I've really hurt myself, Pat. I'm bleeding. I've left the house and come to the station because I'm standing on the platform, and I don't know what to do.
My family is threatening to call an ambulance. I don't know what to do.

I Don't See Much Point to This Anymore

Sophie, if you are in such a bad way then you must listen to them. I am not there with you, and they would not be doing this lightly.
Things are out of hand when you say you are cutting and at the railway.

I've left the house.

Are you safe leaving the house?

I don't know.

Then that's why they are worried and rightly so. If it's a general not coping with the past, then you may need some help.

I feel very very unwell.

Do you need me to ring as I'm very worried about you?

It's too fucking hard and I don't want to rely on anyone. I'm sorry. I don't mean to swear. I'm not swearing at you. I don't know what the hell I'm doing or where I even am.

Do you want a call? It seems all your anger is finally surfacing, only in the form of a tsunami.

I wouldn't know what to say.

You might feel better having human contact? The other thing is it is getting late and if you don't go home, they will call the police.

OK. I'm going home now.

The next morning.

Thank you for last night.

You are very welcome. I hope you are feeling better and that you can find a way forward. Take care and keep me posted. I will be busy until 8 p.m.

I'm not feeling better, sorry. I'm back to working.

Have you and your husband talked about what you should do?

He's asked the GP for some more tramadol.

OK, do you think that will help?

I don't know.

What about a phone call to [the psychiatrist] re antidepressants?

I've still got my antidepressants so I can start again if I choose to.

OK.

He just gets cross and upset and says he doesn't know what to do. I got angry because he threatened to call an ambulance and I don't trust him now.
He can't win whatever he does. It's all my fault.

So how would you like to handle the situation . . . ? Step back from it and see what you would advise a friend in this situation because when things get out of hand it gets frightening and, as you know, everyone handles fear in a different way. If you want to take control, then you must do that, otherwise someone has to intervene. I know you prefer for that not to happen.

I don't know. I need to work, and I haven't got time to go to the hospital.
I need to wait it out and maybe it will pass.

It seems to all build to a head at night when your tolerance is less, so maybe a less punishing work schedule would be better. Maybe your machine broke for a reason!

Everyone is worried about me, and they feel unsafe and because of that I feel guilty but also angry. I can't help who I am and I'm trying, and I'd done it. I'd stopped drinking. I'd stopped harming. I don't need judgement because I judge myself harshly enough. Believe me.

I am not judging you and it is not helpful for you to judge yourself either. Can I suggest that if you have had a drink, go to bed before it releases the anger, and then work through some of the anger the next day? The fact that death was your only answer to the situation shows me how deeply depressed you are.
The concern I have is the outbursts of anger at others, and yourself. The anger seems to be becoming more destructive and an outlet is necessary for it. Alcohol and tramadol are not providing it for you.

**I had a dream the night before last. It felt very important.
I was sitting with my child's nursery school teachers, and I was stressing the importance of [the abuser] not being able to have access to him. In my dream I very clearly said, 'He raped me.'
It is the only time I've heard myself say that so clearly in a dream or in life.**

You see on the one hand you are processing things for the first time and on the other there is too much pain to bear. Then the anger emerges and unfortunately you blame the wrong person . . . You blame yourself for something you couldn't control because you were just a child, and she is left all alone and unsupported as she still is now. Then you punish her some more.
You have come so far with this. Now you must learn to love the child to move out of this web of deceit and destruction.

What deceit?

Childhood pretence that everything was all OK, when, in reality, you lived with a monster and a rapist. Not your deceit. Theirs.

When I just wrote 'raped me' I felt nothing but when I just read your words 'a rapist', the body memory just hit me like a ton of bricks.

So that is what he is – detach from this creature. He is not human.

Pat, it's coming back. I'm so scared.

You have to move around and distract yourself as I am now on my last call of the night. Will talk to you in a while.

I will call you later.

Yes, call me at 10 p.m.

There Is Something Wrong With Me

At this stage in my journey with Pat I was firmly in the camp of 'there is something mentally wrong with me' and was happy to outline with Pat, whose job it was to safeguard at this point, a plan of action that involved possible inpatient care. This never happened because Pat's availability made me feel able to continue processing the trauma at home. What I was creating felt precious and fragile, and with hindsight I know if I had gone into hospital, the chances are I would never have returned to the therapy with Pat. I'm grateful she was there to help me navigate my way through the darkness and to examine the feelings and not to suppress them in the way they would have been in hospital. From experience I know my distress would have been managed there in a very different way – with strong sedatives, sleeping pills or even anti-psychotics. I would have returned home, back to square one and would I have ever tried to access therapy again? Probably not.

To: Sophie
From: Pat
Hi Sophie,
I have received your email and I think this [plan of action] is now a good way forward.
Just to update, I have received [the psychiatrist's] email and note that she acknowledges you have found your voice and you have. You have come such a long way, but you are currently too frightened to look back and see that, and equally too frightened to look ahead.
In the months I have worked with you, you have moved mountains. Now is the time to be still on the summit, and look at the view, and contemplate everything you have had to process. You are so nearly there with this . . . it is like a runner in the last few metres of the race – she knows she's almost there but is feeling exhausted.

Trust the next part of the process.

Your psychiatrist sounds like a nice lady, and you are a very different Sophie – now you know how to speak, and you even used the word on the phone to me yesterday. Stay strong. You can make it because you have a resilient mind.

To: Pat
From: Sophie
Thank you. I don't know what to do.

To: Sophie
From: Pat
Are you able to wait it out for her call on Friday afternoon?

To: Pat
From: Sophie
I am speaking with you on Friday afternoon.
Right now, I feel very disconnected from my body. Like I'm drugged. I'm trying to work but can't get myself going. Meanwhile I'm accepting sewing orders for next week.

To: Sophie
From: Pat
I feel you are driving on and not acknowledging where the road even is. Never mind about speaking to me on Friday . . . speak to [the psychiatrist] first. That is the most important thing because we can catch up at any time. She is offering a way forward. And if you need an admission before then, you have your options. No matter what, now is not a good time to take any more orders. You are physically too unwell to do any more work. How are you managing that and looking after children?

To: Pat
From: Sophie
With my usual competence and aplomb, I expect.
Maybe there's some hope if I can still see humour in this shit.

To: Sophie
From: Pat
Absolutely! You are truly amazing.

To: Pat
From: Sophie
I've agreed to Friday afternoon.

To: Sophie
From: Pat
That's all good, sound reasoning, so well done.

To: Pat
From: Sophie
Thank you. That's what I thought. I'm able to compose a reasonable, unemotional, and measured email, yet I can feel illness raging in my head. I'm like two different people. I know what she's going to want to do. She'll want me to go on to mood stabilisers to control the cycling. What would you do?

To: Sophie
From: Pat
How did this affect you before? What you must consider is . . . are the side effects worse than what you are experiencing by living with what would be considered by some as the illness raging in your head?

To: Pat
From: Sophie
It's one of the few meds for bipolar that I haven't tried.

To: Sophie
From: Pat
OK, so it's unknown. So, see what she says about it.

To: Pat
From: Sophie
It's the hair loss side effect that concerns me. It's not weight gaining.

To: Pat
From: Sophie
Attachment: Picture of chaos of sewing stuff, crochet, materials, yarn
An accurate representation of the inside of my head.

To: Sophie
From: Pat
So, your head certainly needs a rest. You may not necessarily get hair loss . . . It isn't a certain side effect like chemo, and if it begins to happen, they can slowly wean you off and give you something else. You are young so your hair would quickly recover.

To: Pat
From: Sophie
It hasn't recovered from my hair pulling. It's a big problem, hence the worry.

To: Sophie
From: Pat
Well, your hair pulling is different because you are traumatising the scalp continually. If you stopped for several months, it would probably recover.

Fighting the Demon

Around this time, I took part in The Truth Project – a listening exercise, part of The Independent Inquiry into Child Sexual Abuse, set up after the Jimmy Savile Inquiry. It concluded in October 2021 and the IICSA published its final report in October 2022.

This significant step was directly influenced by my therapy. I was sensing that sharing my story might be the way out of the darkness and I wanted it to have meant something. The thought of my experiences being used to influence change intrigued and empowered me to speak out. I reflect often on this time and the juxtaposition between struggling at times to the point of suicidal ideation, and starting what ultimately became my step into the world of activism.

I wonder had I told my contact at The Truth Project what was going on for me, would I have been deemed too vulnerable to take part? This rigidity applies to some rape and sexual abuse support services when wanting to volunteer. I remember enquiring only to be told I could do so two years post the end of the support. I think it's an outdated, paternalistic view with undertones of the innate belief that survivors are 'just too vulnerable'. I believe we should be encouraged to consider using our traumatic experiences as a reason *to* take part in awareness-raising and activism, right from the start. As long as the survivor's involvement is carefully held through robust support then it could be the key to opening the door to healing. Yes, it might be considered risky but the alternative – sending people down the mental health system where our trauma is often suppressed, as it is a system with limited understanding of how to support those with trauma resulting from CSA – is equally risky. People die when under mental health teams in the community and people die on psychiatric wards. Taking part in The Truth Project was my choice and an extremely positive step forward.

> I'm supposed to be doing The Truth Project on Tuesday. Are you free afterwards for an appointment? Instead of this Friday? They suggest to the people that they make contact with their counsellors if they have them. They said it's about an hour to an hour and a half. I do want to do it. I started the process 2 years ago and I had to postpone it a lot because of logistics.

As long as you don't think it will destabilise things further. You can see how you feel on the day.

> OK, thank you so much. Things change so much by the day, sometimes by the hour.

Exactly, so let me know on the day.

Later, that day.

> I'm so frightened of it coming back again. I feel a panic spreading over my body and head and am scared I'm not strong enough to control it. My children have witnessed paramedics in my house before and I can't let this get a grip.

What are you frightened of? . . . What do you mean by it coming back?

> Whatever the fuck is wrong with me. My madness.

OK, have you finished your work and are you in pain?

> I'm still working. Yes, I'm in a lot of pain. I move constantly, you know, like when you're in labour and you can't stay still.

Why can't you take some Tramadol now? It would reduce the pain and relax your mind so you can take some control of this before your call on Friday. If you like . . . relax and discipline the mind even if you must numb it for the moment.

> I can't. I've had a drink and my worst night was on Monday after taking tramadol.

Can you halve the dose or even quarter it if you have had a drink? Does the drink calm or agitate you? If it calms you, I would suggest doing that rather than Tramadol. I am not advocating you take up drinking but in these circumstances, you need to calm yourself until you speak to [the psychiatrist] and begin meds.

It calms my muscles but agitates my mind. It releases an anger inside me that I direct at myself. I am the worst sort of drinker and if this ends and I'm still here, I will return to sobriety like I did before, if I can. The tramadol is slow release so I can't break the tablet.
[The psychiatrist] is keen for me to try a therapy called RTMS that she is now licensed to provide.
But it feels too medical for me to try although it doesn't have the same awful side effects as ECT apparently – mainly memory loss.

I have something for you to think about . . . When a person has experienced the maximum fear, from physical and emotional trauma and has already stepped onto the other side of that fear and lived and felt their anger first rage then subside into acceptance, they will come to see that they have nothing more to fear. Especially if they have a mind like yours that has already learned to fly.

I'm writing more of my story. I don't know where the rage comes from or when it will ever end.

Write it until the forest fire smoulders and the hot embers stop glowing and it becomes ash. The anger is not towards you, it is for the situation you were made to endure.

You Are Never Back Where You Started

Spring

To: Pat
From: Sophie
Hi Pat,
 I'm wondering if we could meet again. I'm really struggling this week, particularly today.
 There is something wrong with me. I can't stop crying. I don't know if I can live in this world anymore.

To: Sophie
From: Pat
Sorry, just picked up, Sophie. I am so, so glad to hear you are crying. I know it is painful, but you are crying again. You can FEEL again and in time you will learn to live again. I hope you pick this message up before you sleep. And yes, you can live in this world, to change it for your children and many others. Your story is so powerful – it must be heard from you.

To: Pat
From: Sophie
I'm in a bad way tonight and it has been building up.

To: Sophie
From: Pat
OK, I understand . . . It's like a dam bursting but once you feel again, you can live again.

To: Pat
From: Sophie
I think I'm a poor mother when I'm like this and I am full of self-hatred for being the way I am. It felt like I was much further on in

the journey, and I'm devastated that I'm now back exactly where I started.

To: Sophie
From: Pat
You are never back where you started. Change is going on all the time. Sliding back temporarily is all part of it until, eventually, as our mutual acquaintances from the groups would say, you get bored with it all. So bored that you are forced to move on and focus and train the mind to be done with the destructive side of abuse. When you realise that you are doing exactly what your abuser hopes you will do – namely, become as dark and destructive as them – then you wake up and question what the hell you are doing . . . namely, destroying yourself for someone who should be locked up. Blaming yourself for the behaviour of an abuser, no matter if they are a family member, just makes no sense at all and is not a sensible coping mechanism . . . In fact, it is the very worst coping mechanism anyone can use, because it is so senseless and unreasonable and provides no room for reasoning at all.

To: Pat
From: Sophie
I truly felt I was at that point. What if it's done such damage to my brain during such a critical stage of development that I can't ever stop, no matter how bored I become of it? I am bored. I'm fed up and bored and tired of all of it.

To: Sophie
From: Pat
With regards to your brain, look on the internet at how much our cells change throughout a year . . . We are renewing them all the time. Change the conditioning and the rigid belief and the body adapts accordingly . . . When you introduce 'possibilities' instead of 'rigidity' a tremendous amount can change – e.g. you were told by an 'expert' that children were not an option for you . . . Well, that was one expert's belief system you shattered!

To: Pat
From: Sophie
Thank you.

Chapter 10

Part Two of his plan he called,

Turning Out the Lights

> But the king said, 'One feather is of no use to me, I must have the whole bird.'
>
> – *The Golden Bird*, The Brothers Grimm

One summer's day, the Little Princess was running in the garden, trying to catch one of the fluff of feather chicks that pecked and darted here and there. They were far too quick for the Little Princess and would peck, hop, flutter out of reach, every time. She laughed when she saw how funny they looked. She tried to catch them because she loved them so much and craved the feel of their tiny warm bodies and their pointy scratchy feet in her gentle hands.

She could see the Evil King crouched on the grass a little way away, with his back to her. She couldn't see what he was doing, and she was curious. She edged a bit closer.

'Come and see,' said the Evil King softly. There, in his giant hands, sat one of the feathered chicks. The Little Princess was delighted. 'Would you like to hold it?' asked the Evil King.

The Little Princess was wary, but the sun was shining, and the Evil King was smiling, so she decided to trust him.

As she reached out to touch the little bird, a huge cloud that hadn't been there before, moved in front of the sun, and the Little Princess felt Icy Cold in the Shadow.

The yellow chick looked at the Little Princess with its bright, beady eyes.

'I'm sorry,' the Little Princess whispered and, in an instant, large and Evil hands, with a violent jerk and twist, snapped the neck of the tiny chick.

The Evil King stood up and tossed the bird on the ground. With a flick of the devil's tail that had appeared behind him, he strode into the depths of the cottage and the Little Princess picked up the still warm just-hatched chick and felt life leave its poor broken body. The lights had gone out in its eyes and the Little Princess understood clearly now.

Click, click, whirr, click went the cameras and the photographs of the Evil King's broad back, the beady black eyes and the *dart, dart, peck* were stacked and shelved neatly in a new box inside her mind labelled, *Turning Out the Lights Day*, and she couldn't get rid of them however hard she tried.

Raindrops fell from the cloud, but the Little Princess realised they were tears. 'Stupid,' she said and hardened her heart a little bit more.

Chapter 11

No-God
Who Art In Heaven

Every man's life is a fairy tale written by God's fingers.

– Hans Christian Andersen

One day, the Little Princess came home from school and the Butterfly Queen sat her down at the kitchen table. She gave her a glass of cold milk and a Custard Cream and told her with a very serious face that she had Some Very Sad News.

The Very Sad News was that her guinea pigs had Got Out. They had escaped from their run and it was very sad but the guinea pigs were not sad. They were having fun and eating dandelions and running in the sky with all the other little guinea pigs. The Butterfly Queen explained that some people called this place in the sky Heaven. The Little Princess was sad, and she cried, but she knew about Heaven as she prayed every day at School to a father called God Who Art In Heaven, and she knew it was a Good place.

A few days later, the Little Princess sat in her secret camp under the lilac bush and cried. She was cross with God for taking her pets and she didn't want to pray to them in Heaven. She wanted to speak to them in the garden and cuddle them and hear their happy squeaks as they nibbled the dandelions she picked for them each day. She wanted her guinea pigs back.

The Evil King, who was never far away, heard her cries and asked the Little Princess what was wrong. He listened to her talk about Heaven and dandelions and God, and it gave him an idea.

The Evil King gently pushed the Little Princess's hair from her damp face. He carefully wiped a tear from her cheek.

'Your guinea pigs are not in Heaven' said the Evil King, and the Little Princess was confused.

'But they Got Out,' she said. 'the Butterfly Queen said so.'

'Yes, that's right, but they didn't go to Heaven because there is no such thing. Do you want to see your guinea pigs?"

And the Little Princess, confused but happy, took hold of the Evil King's large hand.

The Little Princess was surprised when they walked to the bottom of the garden because she'd played there earlier and hadn't seen her guinea pigs. She was surprised when the Evil King grabbed a spade from the vegetable patch. She was surprised when he started digging in the compost heap – a stinking mountain taller than her head of grass cuttings, egg shells, dog shit and worms. She was surprised to see buried deep inside the putrid mound, orange and white tufts of fur and little pink feet. Most of all she was surprised by the maggots. They were everywhere. They wiggled inside bloody holes. They disappeared up pinhole nostrils. They crawled from staring eyes.

The Little Princess watched and watched and listened to the Evil King talk about her little dog and sharp teeth and ripped necks and broken spines and *shaken like rats*. The Little Princess watched and listened as Heaven closed the door and the sun went out and God fell out of the sky

* * *

The next day was Monday. The Teacher told the class to draw a picture. They were to call it What I Did At The Weekend.

The Little Princess sat quietly. Her head hurt and she picked her crayons carefully. She chose orange, pink, black and red and she drew tufts and feet and mountains. She drew a sky with no-Heaven and she drew No-God on the ground. She drew crawling maggots and bloody holes and staring eyes and she handed the picture to The Teacher before going to assembly.

The Little Princess sat in a row and closed her eyes. She did not pray to No-God Who Art In Heaven. She wondered instead why The World could not see Tricks and Traps and why Grown-Ups were so stupid.

Exploring 'No-God Who Art In Heaven'

Is My Darkness Too Much For You?

To: Pat
From: Sophie
Pat, please tell me if this is too much. I don't want to upset you with my story.

To: Sophie
From: Pat
Don't worry, Sophie, I can handle what you are sending me. I am just concerned for you, that you are able to go on handling so much, even though you are detaching from it in this story form. I have such difficulty knowing that someone as evil as he is, is living his life amongst others, without anyone saying a word. This monster is the same as Jimmy Savile . . . a complete predator. I suspect he is doing this with other children too.

To: Pat
From: Sophie
It's strange to hear you say that as my mantra was always that it could have been worse and that others had it worse than me. I just feel numb and detached.

To: Sophie
From: Pat
That's been your way of coping all these years, because if you hadn't had coping mechanisms, you would still be in the psychiatric hospital.

To: Pat
From: Sophie
I'm frightened.

To: Sophie
From: Pat
What are you frightened of?

To: Pat
From: Sophie
I'm not sure. Slipping back maybe. Not being able to fix myself.
Conjuring up the devil.
Sounds ridiculous I know.

When writing these fairy tale chapters, I wrote certain words with capital letters because they were the most important ones of all, reflecting the trauma, or more specifically the darkness of CSA. Some are words loaded with secrets – *Body, Snakes* – others are words that evoked emotion relating to distrust or a power imbalance – *Teacher. Rules. Doctor.* There were the words that reflected self-perception, such as *Shame, Weak, Stupid*, and some of the capitalised words were connected to darkness itself – *Evil. Cold Ice. Shadow of Rocks.* Until I met Pat, the *World* itself felt dark.

As a child at bedtime, I would ask the same questions. *Are there any ghosts? Is it Halloween?* The same words asked night after night. I was frightened – of ghosts, of darkness, a fear of what I couldn't see in the dark and of what might see me. I was frightened Dark would obliterate me and I would disappear. I was faceless in the dark. I was just a body. Sometimes he would come into my bedroom long after the person reassuring me – *no, there are no ghosts. No, it's not Halloween tonight* – had gone downstairs.

The darkness was always on the periphery, waiting to besiege and occupy my mind and it was connected to him. Darkness was living and breathing, and it resided in my house, invisible to everyone else and I had to pretend it was not there at all.

The darkness didn't leave when the abuse ended. I was infected and I personified this absence of light as a devil in my writing, written as a diary entry during this time, and I later included in a blog called *Dance Then, Wherever You May Be*.

My devil is heavy, sitting on my back.
He weighs me down. His foul breath assaults my senses
and fires memories I thought I'd buried. He cheerfully
hands me the spade to dig them up again.
When I'm making a cup of tea, or putting my children to
bed, he pinches my shoulder and puts his evil hands over

my eyes, and I view the world through the gaps in his bony fingers and everything becomes tainted with shadow and filth.
He whispers dark thoughts in my ears. He tells me my happiness isn't real and that it will disappear soon enough. He tells me that by rights, I shouldn't really be here at all, that I should have died.
He flicks his forked tail, and his knees press against my sides and my body memories fire. They're unbearable. They are the unwelcome reminder of where I was touched and what that felt like and my body reacts like it did once again. I'm ready to fight, to run, but I don't. I freeze, like I did back then, and I climb up the stairs, slowly, carefully, like an old woman, crawl under the duvet and close my eyes. If I'm lucky, the devil will sleep when I do. I pray he won't enter my dreams instead.

Child Sexual Abuse feels evil because it *is* an evil act that attacks the body, mind, and soul. Trauma work with Pat was about telling my story but it was about unleashing this darkness into the world. I knew it was irrational but expelling this evil and articulating the words felt dangerous. Selfish, even. At least when the words were unspoken, they were contained. Safe inside me. Once spoken, that darkness was free to travel onwards. What if it latched onto Pat, the recipient of the darkness?

I was beginning to really believe I could live differently but something's gone wrong again in my head. I've fallen down a black hole and I'm struggling. I'm sorry to be that client. I thought I was alright.

Don't worry, Sophie, it's a slip back for a while into the old, frightened way. A small thought for you to dwell on . . . Being 'successful' is the scariest part when you are coming through this. Look at Marianne Williamson's quote from *A Return to Love: Reflections of the Principles of a course in Miracles*. It is the light we are most afraid of particularly when we have lived in the dark.

"Our deepest fear is not that we are inadequate.
Our deepest fear is that we are powerful beyond measure.

It is our light, not our darkness, that most frightens us. We ask ourselves, "Who am I to be brilliant, gorgeous, talented and fabulous?' Actually, who are you not to be? You are a child of God, your playing small doesn't serve the world.
There's nothing enlightened about shrinking so that other people won't feel insecure around you.
We were born to make manifest the glory of God that is within us.
It's not just in some of us; it's in everyone. And as we let our own light shine, we unconsciously give other people our permission to do the same.
As we are liberated from our own fear, our presence automatically liberates others."

I'm struggling to understand memory. Why would I have one clear memory of being 3 and then it ends so abruptly? Why can I even remember what I was wearing but then some memories around 7-9 are intermittent? It's not a traumatic memory so then why block that bit out? None of this makes sense to me today.

Don't spend time trying to do too much. The memories will come back when they are ready to. Sometimes we don't understand the ones that come back because they will seem 'trivial' in comparison to others, but it can be these that carry greater emotional content. As we flow and piece your life together, we don't know what might come.

Thank you. I'm struggling. I'm not sleeping and when I do I have awful nightmares about being trapped and buried alive.

The next day . . .

I'm on the verge of self-harming. I'm really close. It's not just because of the dream but other things too. I'd like to see if telling someone before it happens might help me stop. I also don't want you to feel any responsibility for the outcome. I'm fully responsible for everything I do.

Sophie, can you keep messaging to relieve it? I have a client for an hour and then I can call you. Just keep up a dialogue with me by texting.

Pat and I spoke for few hours via text.

Be angry at the monster not you.
Write down your anger at the perpetrator.

My anger is at [the perpetrator].

OK, don't do anything you will regret. You are in control of this now.

I'm trying to be in control. [My husband and I have argued] but he doesn't know what else is going on in my head of course. It's not his fault that he doesn't know. It's just the way it is.

Walk away telling him this row is taking you to a bad place in the past where you don't want to be. Deep breaths and no need to hurt you because you have argued. You are now in control and arguing is part of life.

Yes, it is. It feels too much when my mind is heavy.

OK, breathe deeply and let the mind also breathe, let the tightness slowly release.

I'm so sorry, Pat.

If you have confronted a monster in the past and survived, why should you not survive again?

**Because I've been half dead since he did what he did. It's not about survival, it's about healing. Coming back to life.
There are only so many times you can confront a monster.
Thank you for everything. I have not self-harmed, but I have now eaten and can't keep it inside me as it sits like a stone.**

Small steps, yes?

And you are gradually doing that. If you weren't you wouldn't be able to argue or get angry. Part of returning to life is being red and fiery. Sometimes it burns out of control for a while, but that's necessary until it can burn steadily, bright, and beautiful again. When you have confronted a monster enough times, he no longer returns because you have learnt how to slay him. You might want something small to eat as you need to keep your immune system tip top. From little acorns big oak trees grow!

I've always been fiery! I see red and explode. But I learned to turn it inwards unfortunately.

Now turn it out and let it burn.

My stone still sits within me, but I haven't thrown it up or self-harmed. That's an achievement, isn't it?

That is wonderful. Well done to you, under such difficult circumstances also. You did it. Tonight, you DID achieve NOT going back to old coping mechanisms.

Dream Telling

To: Pat
From: Sophie
Subject: Dreaming
I dreamed my old school became my home.

    I was house sitting in my family home and looking after the dogs when I got a job as a receptionist at the school. I wanted this job and was so happy with my first day. I felt like I had achieved something very important. My husband and children came after the day ended because I had things to do, and he put them in a bedroom that was in the school because it was getting late, and later I wanted to go to bed too and was exhausted. I knew the dogs had been alone and shut in all day with no food so I had to go back but I couldn't because I was so tired. I thought I'd try and sleep at school and get up at 5 a.m. instead but then I overslept. There was a constant pull and feeling of guilt.

    There was also a threatening feeling at night, again. I was walking the corridors and the stairs, and I knew we weren't alone. There was a caretaker. I could hear his music from another part of the school, so I searched for where it was coming from and ended up looking through a crack in a door and seeing a man in the bath. I retreated and feared he'd sensed me there. I knew there were no locks on any of the doors and I felt unsafe. The room that was my new 'bedroom' was my old history classroom. As I looked at the bed, I knew I would be raped on it by the caretaker. It was inevitable.

To: Sophie
From: Pat
Let's look at this dream bit by bit. First, we have the school which clearly meant a lot to you in the dream . . . It became your 'home' – and this would suggest a place of safety on some level. You have [your family home and the animals] again and your pull between them and the work you had to do at school. What was this important 'work' at the school about?

    There is a feeling of guilt. The children were sleeping at the school, again a 'safe' place. You had a plan, but then you overslept and couldn't complete your plan. Over sleep tends to make one think that, deep down, there was a desire not to action a plan, and by over sleeping there was also an excuse for not completing the task. What does this task of not feeding the dogs mean to you? Now we go to the 'caretaker', an interesting choice of words and this feeling of him sensing you there. He was also in the bath, so you were aware of him without his clothes on. Think also about the bathroom in your 'real' home. You know that there were no locks on the doors . . . nowhere was safe. The history room which is now your bedroom certainly isn't safe. What does the history room mean to you? What did it mean to you when you were younger?

The final and important thing in all of this was you have finally used the word rape and you have been able to say, 'I knew I would be raped on the bed by the caretaker. It was INEVITABLE.' Your mind is getting ever closer to telling you. This caretaker in charge of the whole school, when no one else was there, was preparing himself in the bathroom having removed his clothes to do what was inevitable.

Now piece it together, Sophie. In your words, answer the questions I have asked. How amazing are dreams that process things for us even when we are asleep? How amazing was the psychologist who discovered the importance of dreams? And even more amazing, is this truly extraordinary client that has come into my life. Take care of yourself.

To: Pat
From: Sophie
Some images are constantly coming into my mind today. I can't tell what is the dream and what isn't. I feel like something has unlocked a bit and I'm needing more.

There's one image that keeps coming into my mind. From the dream . . . Do you think that means it's more likely what that image shows did happen? Or is it just a horrible image from the dream?

To: Sophie
From: Pat
If it's horrible and is being revealed, write it, or draw it. Detaching all emotions from it as if it is a picture from a film or one you have come across on Pinterest.

To: Pat
From: Sophie
OK. Then what do I do with it?

To: Sophie
From: Pat
Either send a picture in email as a photoshot or email what you have written so that you give it to me and release it from you. You have then validated it, shared it, and taken some of the burden away from it.

I shared with Pat an image of myself in a certain position that was persistently coming back to me in flashbacks and in dreams.

To: Sophie
From: Pat
I have picked up your email, so you have now 'released' this to me. Remain calm and composed as anything else flows. Remember none of whatever happened to you has anything to do with 'You'. It is a depraved monster that was in your life, and as you get stronger you will slay him in your chosen way.

To: Pat
From: Sophie
So why have I not seen this particular image before? I've always been on my back for the darkest memories.
    And why do I now feel like rewinding and not sending you that email? It makes no sense.

To: Sophie
From: Pat
Just leave the photos as they are and let the memories settle. Don't question them and feel no tension in having sent them. They are what has been given to you today. We don't know what the darkest memories really are, but at the moment the unconscious is releasing things. Just let it do that without too much judgement about them.

At this stage I had more knowledge than Pat thought. I knew

how *bad* it had been but had pushed away memories as they surfaced and never acknowledged to myself just how bad. Dreams and flashbacks were very distressing, and processing difficult because it put the memories under a spotlight. I think deep down I was looking for a way out. Maybe if Pat had said, *these are just dreams, they mean nothing*, I could put my knowledge back behind the Big Black Door and pretend nothing had happened to me. I'm glad Pat allowed me to bring the dreams into my work and didn't disregard them. Discussing them with Pat gave me permission to *say it* without actually having to say it.

It made me feel vulnerable to share my story. Recently I worked with an academic who told me of a clever way she highlights the enormity of sharing secrets, when teaching students about trauma. She asks them to write a secret on a piece of paper and then collects the pieces of paper, putting them in a bag. She asks the students how it makes them feel, knowing she has their secret. *Scared*, they say and, *Regretful. I don't know what you're going to do with it*. They express relief when she throws the bag away at the end of the lecture. I was handing Pat my secrets and trusting she wouldn't let me down. Once words are spoken, they can't be taken back, but sharing my story through emails and messages gave me an element of control. Sometimes I'd ask Pat to delete a message or email. She would do this without question. This helped to build trust and my need for Pat to do this lessened as we went along.

Do you mind deleting the pictures I sent you yesterday?

No, that's fine. I can delete them.
Done.

Thank you. Sorry.

No need to be sorry. You have complete control of this journey – do what feels comfortable for you.

I just can't comprehend that particular image and therefore I can't trust it.

> If you can't comprehend it and you can't trust it, just leave it in the book 'as a return to later image' in case any other images come through.

> **Yes, I need to. Processing that is something I can't do in messages. I need human contact and touch. It helped me before when I was with you in that session as I felt without it like a helium balloon about to float away. To just be able to reach out for you made me feel safer.**

> That's why I suggested filing it because you need human contact to help you process some things.

And then came the question I had been desperately wanting to ask. I asked it because I *needed* Pat to say yes. If she did, I felt it would give me permission to say the words.

> **Do you think I was raped?**

> In answer to your question, given the extent of the monster you lived with, I think it is highly likely. Also given the extent of your trauma response, it would also be highly indicative that you were. As you process this, you must have a strong mind and remember whatever this gross monster did, he did not and never will destroy you. Focus now on your plans for the future and all the women you are going to take forward with you.

> **Am I not allowed to feel the horror and grief of it? If I do, then am I not being strong enough? Or is my mind not strong enough? What if I need to focus on what happened , rather than the future? What if I allow myself to feel the hurt and begin to heal before looking to the future?**

> As long as the truth doesn't overwhelm you. Sometimes when the truth suddenly hits you, it can go either way. You can gradually understand why you behaved as you did and understand yourself and give yourself the compassion and love you deserve as well as grieving for the loss, or it can

send you reeling and spinning, and it can overpower you. You must do what is best for you. Sometimes if you have a goal, especially one to help others, it can help you to help yourself. You have a purpose and a will to live. As I once said, find a purpose and a will to live and you will come through this and not regret who you are. You have yet to understand how truly amazing you are.

I'm not ready to look forward until I look at what happened.

OK, then look at what happened and keep me on board, that way you won't go into harming. We both must trust you are ready to process the next extent of this horror.

Moving Mountains

I don't need you to delete these chapters but please can you give me some feedback when you're able to? Old habits die hard, don't they, and just sharing it with you makes me feel the shame of it. I'm wondering if your take on this would help me to alleviate that particular emotion. If not, I may need it deleted. You must think I'm totally bonkers. I'm being as honest with you about this as I can possibly be. Thank you.

Good morning, Sophie. I am working for the moment on a project for a few hours and then when I need a break, I will give you feedback. I don't think you are bonkers at all. You need clarification and validation of what went on. Meanwhile it would be interesting for you to do some research on psychopathy and the traits of narcissistic personality disorder. Not sharing became a coping mechanism for you, because as you said, 'you just knew not to say anything'.

There is an email on its way . . . The chapters are coming thick and fast at the moment.

OK, thank you. I will catch up later, and well done. It sounds as though things are flowing again which is great news. Your mental health seems better when this is happening.

There I have sent it. It's called Rules.

Excellent. You are as busy as me!

I expect you're dressed though . . . I'm still in my pyjamas.
I'm not, but I again have muddy trousers from this morning's walk!

Please can you delete the last one? Called Rules. I have edited it and need it to be just right.

I have sent you back an email on the first one. I will of course delete the last one. I hope my explanation in the email will clarify your reactions in many situations given such abject cruelty. I will say it again . . . how you have come out of this the way you have leaves me in awe. His cruelty and sickness knew no boundaries.

I'm going to send you the edited version now. Is that OK?

Yes. Send me back any comments on my email.

I've just sent Rules – part two. I can't seem to stop.

OK, thank you for your emails. I will comment on them later tonight.

Later . . .

Have you read all my emails or just that first one?

All of them.

Are you able to give me more feedback? The Lay-by one is bothering me. I don't mean tonight. Thank you for your replies today.

Stay in those PJs, no guilt, don't worry about a thing because you are moving mountains in your room!

Chapter 12

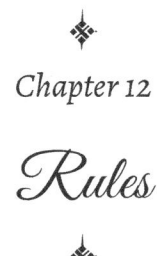

Rules

Her tender feet felt as if cut with sharp knives, but she cared not for it; a sharper pang had pierced through her heart.
  – The Little Mermaid, Hans Christian Andersen

The Evil King was bored.

He enjoyed hurting the Little Princess very much. He loved to taste her Fear and craved more of it, but he was bored of how Good the Little Princess was, how quickly she Obeyed his orders.

The Evil King decided he needed to make it harder for her, so he went to his shed and consulted his Big Black Book.

He turned to the chapter called Rules 101 and absorbed himself for a couple of hours, writing notes here and there.

Then one morning, he summoned the Little Princess.

'We will go for a walk,' said the Evil King. They put on their wellingtons and they fastened the lead on the little dog's collar, and he held the Little Princess's hand tightly as they began their journey.

The Little Princess was silent and watchful, and her little hardening heart fluttered inside her chest.

By and by, the little dog, excited to be on a walk and keen to run free in the fields and follow the scent of rabbits in the woods, started to strain and pull against the lead. The Evil King gave the lead a jerk and the dog fell back in line, just like the Little Princess who was walking silently alongside the Evil King. Soon enough, the little dog pulled again, and again the Evil King jerked the lead – a bit harder this time.

The Little Princess was worried. She wanted to warn her little dog to Obey but the little dog wasn't listening. She only cared about long grass and woods and rabbits. She didn't understand about dangerous kings.

The Evil King stopped walking.

'Get me a stick,' he said to the Little Princess. So the Little Princess, with Fear in her heart and the Shadow pulling on her legs, looked around. She saw a thick short stick and picked it up.

The Evil King shook his head. 'Thinner, longer,' he said.

And the Little Princess looked around until she saw a thinner and longer stick. She gave it to the Evil King. He swiped the stick through the air and the Little Princess felt cold in the Shadow that had covered the sun.

'Perfect,' said the Evil King.

They carried on with their walking and the little dog began her frantic pulling.

The Little Princess looked at her little dog. 'I'm sorry,' she whispered, and watched as the Evil King raised the stick in the air and, with a vicious swipe, landed it down on the little dog's nose. The little dog yelped and danced and cowered at the end of her lead and the Evil King smiled.

On they went. The little dog walked back in line next to the Evil King. By and by the little dog began to pull and another cutting blow landed on her nose.

'She has to learn The Rules,' said the Evil King.

Why won't you learn? the Little Princess whispered in her heart to her little dog.

'Now it's your turn,' said the Evil King and he gave the stick to the Little Princess.

The Little Princess was frightened to say no. She gave a tentative tap to the little dog's nose.

'Harder,' said the Evil King.

So the Little Princess tried again.

'Harder,' said the Evil King and his Cold Ice Eyes locked onto her warm brown eyes.

She kept trying and failing and trying and failing until the whip whistled and the Evil King was satisfied. The dog cowered and danced and yelped and the Little Princess wanted to die.

'Good,' said the Evil King. 'You're teaching her not to break The Rules.'

And the Little Princess understood exactly. They continued

with their walk and the Little Princess and her little dog fell in line with the Evil King. He was glad. Falling in line meant they wouldn't be whispering secrets over the Kingdom walls.

That night, whilst the Little Princess was eating her supper, the little dog sat against her legs and the Little Princess put one hand down to stroke her soft black head. The little dog licked the Little Princess's hand over and over and the Little Princess wondered why the little dog would still love such a stupid, Weak and Cowardly girl.

Chapter 13

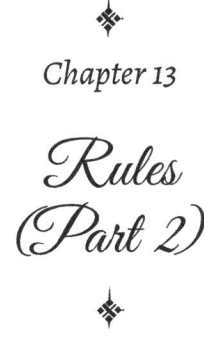
Rules (Part 2)

The good little sister cut off her own tiny finger, fitted it into the keyhole, and succeeded in opening the lock.

– The Seven Ravens, The Brothers Grimm

After the walk, the Evil King spoke to his family. He presented them with a list of Rules. The list was tied up with a red velvet ribbon and he told them, whilst looking at each one in turn with his Cold Ice Eyes, that they must study this list of Rules and learn each and every Rule and to never ever Break The Rules.

The Little Princess couldn't raise her head to look at the Evil King and her head and eyes felt heavy.

She felt his hand under her chin and the Evil King lifted her head for her.

'Do you understand?' he said quietly.

The Little Princess felt cold and her small hardening heart fluttered in her chest. 'Yes,' she whispered, and she took the list away to study.

The list read:

Rules. Particularly important for car journeys.
No shouting.
No fighting.
No arguing.
No laughing.
No singing.
No eating in the car.

No drinking in the car.
No car sickness.
No whistling.
No chewing gum.
No eating sweets.
No music.
No opening the windows.

And the Little Princess breathed a sigh of relief. *How hard can that be?* she wondered. *I can do that.*

But she found that abiding by The Rules was harder than she thought.

One day, the Evil King, the Butterfly Queen and the two Princesses travelled in their car to a place far, far away. On the car journey, the princesses were excited to see the sea and they chattered and planned and laughed and played and the Evil King sat silent in his driving seat. Eventually of course, the laughter was too loud, and the Evil King told them to 'Stop!'

But the excitement of this adventure made the little princesses giggle and poke one another and sing and play and eventually, of course, the Evil King reminded them of The Rules and told them that they had Broken The Rules.

The Princesses fell silent. The Little one blamed the Big, and the Big blamed the Little.

'It's your fault,' they said to each other. 'I hate you,' they reminded each other, and they stopped their laughter and their chatter and their play.

But it was too late. The Evil King's serpent of rage had risen and he was furious. They had Broken The Rules and had to be reminded.

The Little Princess watched as the Evil King twisted around in his seat, his hands flailing wildly, trying to hit and hurt. The Little Princess could see his fury and could see the danger as their car began to veer, this way and that. The more he reached and the more he missed, the angrier he became, and the Little Princess knew they would surely die.

She quickly unbuckled her seatbelt and edged closer to the Evil King until, with great relief, she felt him hit her little bare legs.

She closed her eyes and gritted her teeth and made herself

stay within his reach, until finally the Evil King's anger diminished, and the serpent of rage shrank back to hide within his dead heart.

The car steadied and the journey continued. When the Little Princess was sure the Evil King was facing the right way, she edged back to her seat and buckled her seatbelt.

She saw the Big Princess looking at her and she decided at that moment she wouldn't cry. She would *never* cry again. She pulled her skirt over her red legs so she couldn't see them and looked out of the window and her heart hardened a little bit more.

Exploring 'Rules'

To: Pat
From: Sophie
I'm reading back what I have written and am overwhelmed by the level of psychological abuse. There is so much, yet I always thought it was the lesser evil. Now I can see it was actually the precursor. The sexual abuse took over once the psychological abuse had done its damage and secured my silence.

I have always seen the sexual abuse as worse than the psychological, with the physical being far less of an issue, but now I'm not so sure.

To: Sophie
From: Pat
I think it was all compounded together. The psychological wears away your mind and sense of self, the physical carries the pain in the body and the sexual takes away the soul, resulting in an abuse of mind, body and spirit which is ultimately the essence of a human being. The more you read, the more you will understand and come to realise that this behaviour of his was no different to what the Nazis did in the death camps.

When I next spoke with Pat, she told me she had been for a walk with her dog. By sheer coincidence it was to the same common near to where I had grown up – a place I had been taken to on many occasions by the abuser.

> Just been on a long hike for 3 hours so will read [the next fairy tale chapter] when I get home.
>
> **I'm feeling a bit uncomfortable about you going there and need to just be honest with you and say it. Think I need a bit of reassurance.**
>
> What did you want to say?

Exploring 'Rules'

It's because of where you were. Some of the abuse happened [there]. I spent lots of time there. I was there every day. The thought of you coming across [family members] makes me feel uncomfortable. I don't know why. Sorry.
I'm sorry.
Not sure why it would make me feel uncomfortable. Crazy, right?

No, it maybe just feels strange to you that I live near your old home.

I'd never given it any thought until today.
Can we move on? Wish I hadn't said anything. I am sorry. You don't need to justify anything.

A little while later I messaged Pat again.

Hi, Are you still happy for me to send you more of the story?

Yes, keep it flowing.

Thank you. I've sent it by email.
Please can you let me know when you've read it?

I have sent you an email back.

To: Pat
From: Sophie
Subject: The Common
Dear Pat
I am sorry for my knee jerk reaction yesterday. I had been writing about the place that you told me you went to, and the coincidence made me feel uneasy. When I recall these memories, it's as if I am there.
    It is as if you were 'there' before I was ready to tell you. This place was really an extension of my garden, so it was as if you'd said that you'd taken your dog to walk around my childhood home.

> Of course, you couldn't have known that, and I apologise for questioning you about it.
> Sophie

Pat telling me where she had walked with her dog ended up being quite fortuitous. Therapists might be taught to hold themselves at arm's length, but Pat chooses to work differently. I am grateful she chose to work intuitively with me, not afraid of the dreaded 'boundary crossing' because it opened conversations we might never have had. I shared *The Common* as a direct result of this conversation, which gave Pat a greater understanding of the trauma I was dealing with. I had the opportunity to process it. Was she stepping over boundaries or was she in fact reaching into my world? She reached me in a way no one before had cared to try. It was more than a job to her, and I sensed that.

Chapter 14

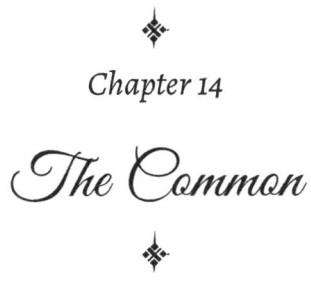

Most of the people who will walk after me will be children, so make the beat keep time with short steps.

– Hans Christian Anderson

Often, the family left The Kingdom of His and went for long walks on The Common. In the puddles of cracked ice and frozen mud of bitter winter, in the wood-smoky, red-brown crunch of autumn, in the bright and startling green of summer and in the Little Princess's favourite season of all, springtime – her birthday month of white snowdrops, daffodils and fresh air, when everything felt brand new.

When she was very small, the Evil King would throw her onto his shoulders and grip her ankles tightly and sometimes, as he strode with purpose across The Common, the top of his head would hit the Little Princess's chin, cracking her teeth together and making her eyes water. She *wouldn't cry* though because she knew he would grip even harder, and her feet would throb. She liked being high up and close to the branches and the sky, but she didn't like being gripped. Sometimes the Evil King would place her in a rusty metal wheelbarrow, next to a heavy axe, and bumpety-bump her along the paths, where they would search for fallen trees and chop them into logs for the fire, or tall sticks for the runner beans.

As she got bigger and her legs grew stronger, the Little Princess would walk by herself. She never complained when she got tired. She was stoic and tough and loved her walks on The Common.

She knew every path and puddle and nook and cranny. She

had her favourite bits – The Cricket Pitch, The Pond with the water boatmen and darting newts, The Bendy Tree, The Gnome Tree – but she had places that she liked less, in the Shadows.

One day on a walk, she was alone with the Evil King. They walked in silence and then the Evil King darted off the path and the Little Princess was confused to see him pull down his trousers and squat in the undergrowth.

'What are you doing?' she asked. She was frightened that someone might see and kept looking all around her just in case.

'I'm desperate,' said the Evil King. 'Watch.'

So, the Little Princess edged closer, peering to see what he was doing. Her eyes and nose were assaulted in the same instant by the rotting stench and image of a brown, shining turd emerging from the Evil King, and the Little Princess clapped her hands over her mouth and stumbled back.

'Stay,' demanded the Evil King. 'Watch me.'

And the Little Princess had no choice. She walked slowly back and stood nearby and watched.

The Evil King watched her watching him and the Little Princess could feel the Cold Ice and she could also see how happy he was, and she didn't understand.

It was A Trick, of course, but she wasn't sure about this one at all. She thought he looked quite stupid, with his Ugly willy hanging down in the leaves and sticks, and she knew he couldn't do much to hurt her when he was over there like that. However, the sky had turned dark and the air felt cold and the Little Princess felt very frightened. She just didn't know what she was frightened of.

'I need to clean myself,' said the Evil King. 'Find me some leaves so I can clean myself.'

So, the Little Princess with her pitter patter heart, picked up a fistful of leaves from by her feet.

'Show me,' said the Evil King.

The Little Princess walked very slowly towards the Evil King, trying not to breathe and showed him the leaves in her hand.

The stench was overwhelming, and the Little Princess couldn't help but gag.

The Evil King smiled. 'Those are no good,' he said, standing up, with his trousers still around his ankles and his Ugly willy hanging for anyone to see.

 The Little Princess looked and checked and quickly grabbed a different type of leaf – a greener, fresher type of leaf for the Evil King to wipe his Ugly, stinking self.

 'Good girl,' said the Evil King and he cleaned himself up, pulled up his trousers and took hold of the Little Princess's hand. Together, they carried on with their walk.

 Click, click, whirr, click, went the cameras in her head and the photographs stacked themselves neatly into a new box labelled, *Shitting in The Woods Day.*

Exploring 'The Common'

To: Sophie
From: Pat
Subject: Re: The Common
Hi Sophie
Please don't feel the need to apologise to me. I don't realise that I am triggering you. He is so, so disgusting, Sophie, one cannot even imagine what it must be like to live inside his head. He is so twisted and dark and evil and gross.

I would so love to see you come through this and find a way to live a wonderful life, rid yourself of his filthy memories and go out there and make a difference, so that eventually his behaviour is known about, without it causing any harm to you. He is so revolting, Sophie. I cannot believe that other children have not been involved. There is no way that when you stopped seeing him, that he has not done this to others. Keep writing and sending them over as you feel ready. Are you feeling any calmer today?

To: Pat
From: Sophie
I moved away when I was 19 and when I was pregnant at 21, I moved 'home' to the countryside where I grew up as I thought I had to bring up a child in the countryside as I had been brought up. We moved to a very pretty cottage with lots of space but the second I shut the door after the removal men left, I felt the beauty of the house had tricked me. I could hear at all times the sound of the traffic (it was on a busy road) and the motorbikes as they raced up and down the road. It was like being back in a lay-by he used to take me, and I had some sort of a breakdown, I think. My husband would go to work, and I would have days and days where I lost myself entirely. I lost hours of time, and we moved 4 months later, when I was 7 months pregnant, to another rural but noisy street, which wasn't much better. I craved the town, and I couldn't bear to live there. I spent many days walking and walking, heavily pregnant, up into [the common] and revisiting the place where I had spent so much of my time, again losing time and 'coming to' hours later. My daughter was born, and we moved as soon as we possibly could, back to a town where I had been happy before

moving back [to the country]. I thrive when I exist in a crowd, surrounded by people. I must see the town because I feel safer in a crowd of people than I do walking in the countryside and woods.

To: Sophie
From: Pat
Everything you are remembering about him is making you realise just how disgusting he is in every way. Eventually you will sit and say this monster is the most disgusting person that ever lived, and you will say that at the end of your story.

To: Pat
From: Sophie
I don't know what I'm frightened of. But I feel really scared.

To: Sophie
From: Pat
Scared maybe that you could get well and all of what happened to you is true and you are validating it and you have survived . . . and as you become powerful, then what . . .? All of this is very scary when you have been so used to being a victim.

To: Pat
From: Sophie
No. That's unfair.

To: Sophie
From: Pat
No, it's true . . . It is every survivor's biggest fear, because you don't know how to be those things.
   It's really scary, because you realise that if you have survived all this, you have such power and if you release it, what do you do with it?

To: Pat
From: Sophie
I'm scared of the fact that I can't breathe properly. I'm scared that I'm being crushed slowly to the point of not being able to breathe at all. I'm scared of having the opportunity to have surgery to stop this. I'm scared of not being able to have surgery because I'm so fucking scared of being touched.

So, I do think that's unfair. I'm different. I'm dealing with this disability too.

And I'm angry.

To: Sophie
From: Pat

OK, so begin by learning to breathe properly by deep belly breaths and exercise every day. Start to build body and mind so you can take on board the next fear. Use that anger to breathe in and out like a dragon breathing fire. By the time you are breathing fire, you will command how you will be touched and by whom.

Eventually the anger at the abuse will reach a crescendo until the respect you want and deserve will come your way because you will settle for nothing else.

How do you want to deal with the disgusting, revolting monster? That is the question.

So, maybe gather the anger and channel it into what you want to do now... your activism, writing the book. He is getting older... he thinks everyone is either mentally ill, is suffering from amnesia due to trauma, too frightened to say a word, or he doesn't even care at all because he thinks everyone else in the world is nothing but pond life.

What he doesn't know is this: there is someone about to emerge from the closet, someone who is much cleverer and more powerful than him, because she walks with truth and knows *exactly* what he is.

Fragments

Summer

To: Pat
From: Sophie
Subject: Lay-by
I need to separate these memories of events into FACT and PROBABLE.
My memories are disjointed, and I picture myself as a little bird, trapped in a cage and see the car from different perspectives which change rapidly as I try to recall this memory in full.
FACT: I remember driving down into the lay-by and this surprised me as it wasn't usual.
FACT: I remember looking up at the cars passing by and seeing them pass behind the trees.
He abused me in the car. I remember the smell of his body and the sensation of being choked and feeling suffocated and hot, but it is not a clear memory like the ones in the bath.
It is probable that he penetrated my mouth.
Is this rape?

To: Sophie
From: Pat
This would be oral rape.

To: Pat
From: Sophie
Thank you.
Please can you delete those emails?

To: Sophie
From: Pat
Of course.

**To: Pat
From: Sophie**
Thank you. I can't explain why that is important, but it leaves me feeling very vulnerable knowing they're there.

**To: Sophie
From: Pat**
I understand completely. It is very important that the person you entrust to take you on such a personal journey does not leave you feeling vulnerable.

**To: Pat
From: Sophie**
I need to get over this hump and then I'll relax a bit.

**To: Sophie
From: Pat**
I understand how difficult it is to trust another person with the very core of your being. That person must earn the client's trust and that sometimes can only be slowly and surely, as part of the journey. We are both on this journey and it is like a mountain climb. The leader of the climb must be sure footed and trustworthy; only then can others make the climb. The leader must constantly check their fitness and ability, and this happens when they challenge and question themselves every day. Every person I work with keeps me in that situation. If I don't do that, then I can't give my best.

Fragments – the shape of a jawline, the smell of cigarettes and whisky on someone's breath. The click of a man's shoes as he walks behind on the street. Being followed up a flight of stairs. A clearing of the throat. A wink. A song on the radio.

When abuse ends, we have to find a way to live with the triggers.

We can all experience flashbacks. They are a pull-back in time to a snapshot of our lives. They're not always bad. The cry of seagull can take us back to a family holiday and sandy ham sandwiches on a beach. The smell of tomatoes can take us back to preparing a salad with a beloved grandmother on a long-forgotten summer's day. A flashback for someone who has suffered abuse is different. It's not a gentle or comfortable reminiscing. At best it is mildly distasteful and at worst it can feel like a violent assault on the senses. Like a kick in the stomach leaving you doubled over, unable to catch your breath. It results in a heightened awareness of the world around us. It takes your body hostage and there's not much you can do about it other than wait for it to pass.

I would describe these as torturous; more than flashbacks, they are *body memories*. These were the cause of great anguish at this point in my life, at times triggering extreme self-harming behaviour in a desperate attempt to shut them down, to cut them out.

It was the pressure on my wrist from an invisible hand.

It was the feeling of my pulse as the pressure built. It was rubbing at my skin to ease the feeling, but that didn't work because there was nothing there at all, just a memory.

It was feeling mental torment as the most intimate parts of me began to remember too. It was relentless and felt so real but there was no one there, no hand, no man. Just a ghost.

Every sense was affected. I had impressions of touch, of smell. I felt pressure and pain. I heard sounds. I saw images in my mind that would play over and over again. I would then relive them in my dreams too. My body would react as if it was under attack – my heart would race, I could feel myself 'leaving' my body, sounds would become more distant – I would feel like I was the other side of a glass wall, that my body didn't belong to me. At its worst, I would feel as if I wasn't even there at all. After one particularly triggering event, I felt like I'd died. Even though my body was still breathing and eating, speaking, moving, I wasn't in it. It was the most frightening and surreal thing to experience.

As I worked with Pat, the flashbacks and body memories worsened. Had I spoken to a psychiatrist about this instead of her, no doubt I would have been given a label of some sort. I would probably have been told I needed medication, to fix the part of my brain that was chemically imbalanced.

Thankfully I had Pat to turn to who told me that what I was experiencing was *normal*. It was a *part of the process*. Not to fear it but to *face it instead*.

So that's what I did. I didn't really have much choice. It was either ride the wave or drown in it and I didn't want to drown. I wanted to be free, and I wanted to live.

Later, I found a method that worked quite well for me. When

I identified a trigger I would write it down. Some were easier to list. But each phrase or word was painfully hard to write. Each one would fire body memories that I wanted to cut out of me, but I carried on and wrote everything that had ever triggered these body memories, however small, until there was nothing more to write.

Then began the 'tracing back to source'. What was the story behind each one?

Some, like the ones below, were straightforward and easier to trace back than others. These ones I could do on my own.

> Trigger: the smell of a certain type of alcohol.
> Cause: It was on his breath when he abused me.
>
> Body memory: Smell/taste/pressure on my body.
> Feeling evoked: depression/fear/dissociation.

Others were so difficult that I chose to work with Pat, in a place where I felt supported and safe. But in physically writing the words down, the triggers began to lose a bit of their power.

I found myself analysing the body memories rather than going into a blind panic. I would remind myself of the trigger, the cause, the body memory, and the feeling. This analysis gave me a focus. It was a way of taking back control. It was like saying to my brain, 'Before you panic, let's just remember where this comes from. Let's give this a bit of thought. This is why your body feels like this. This was the event that caused it. This is in the past. This isn't now. If the body memories want to come, let them, and then let them go.'

The next email described 'memories' I had assumed would stay behind the Big Black Door because they were different to the others. They weren't whole – more intrusive flashes of information. Broken and shocking pieces of reality. I left out these fragmented parts of my story initially because it was always paramount that I document only what I knew for sure was accurate and complete recall. This stems from my early fear of not being believed; if I included anything that could cast doubt on my story then I'd risk the disbelief of others. Many survivors are not believed by their families. Some will stand up in court and tell their story only to be accused of being a fantasist and a liar. I wanted to keep these fragments to myself because I knew

I'd find it hard to cope with not being believed but I knew I'd have to talk about these with Pat. They were festering inside me, and they were making me unwell.

Opening the Big Black Door

To: Pat
From: Sophie
The problem with this chapter is that I haven't got clear memories. I wrote it in the best way I could to describe the feelings I get when I try to recall that event.

Some things are very clear. The cars above and the lay-by itself – after all, I have always known exactly which lay-by this is and have driven past it hundreds of times in my life, holding my breath and not looking every single time. I would feel sick, and my heart would race.

When I did drive there, to try and recall what happened, my memory of the view from the car, the noise from the traffic above was exactly as I remembered it. But then panic takes over and obviously he didn't actually 'chase' me around the car, how could he? Yet my snapshot of memories, which are fleeting, are all from different viewpoints from within the car. The Shadow, the Cat and Mouse, the Snakes all illustrate this feeling of total panic and powerlessness, and the body memories are of feeling hot, choked, totally trapped and completely alone in some awful hell, with someone who I not only feared, but loved too.

To: Sophie
From: Pat
I think you are absolutely right to find your way to put back control. As your therapist it is my duty of care to ensure you're able to manage the horrific things you are having to process, and to support your wishes in this. You are in control now, of your therapy, your self-care and your future.
Keep sending me your writing. Remember to take breaks, put it away for a while when you need to and then come back to it.

I will be working again for a few hours but will pick up in between breaks.

I replied to The Lay-by last night. I think you have to accept what you suspect happened, did happen. Don't forget you may not fully have had the words as a child to understand what he was doing, if this was the first time it occurred.

Chapter 15

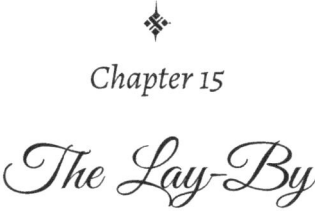

'Once you lose yourself, you have two choices: find the person you used to be, or lose that person completely."

– H. G. Wells

The Little Princess and the Evil King were leaving for The World. As she watched him prepare, the Little Princess saw how clever his disguise was. Although he was tall and handsome on the outside, the Little Princess could sense the Ugly seething and twisting under the surface of his skin. Even though he used the finest colognes, she could smell the rotten stench of Ugly emanating from his festering soul. The Evil King needed the best clothes to cover the Ugly. Only the finest fabrics made by the best tailors and the most expensive shoes made from polished mirrors would do. The Evil King liked to look in his mirrored shoes and admire his Cold Ice Eyes.

The rings on his fingers disguised and tethered The Snakes that the Little Princess would sometimes catch a glimpse of. The Kind and Gentle Mask was undoubtedly the most important of all the disguises. The Little Princess saw it was a Magic Mask and when he placed it very carefully on his face, it made the seething Ugly settle and the rotten smell recede. So powerful was the magic of the Kind and Gentle Mask that even she could forget he was the Evil King if she remembered not to look at the Cold Ice Eyes.

The Little Princess found herself looking forward to these visits to The World. Like everyone else, she thought the Evil King looked fine in his handsome clothes and mirrored shoes and felt proud to be the Little Princess.

One day, they travelled in the car. The Little Princess felt calm and happy to be with the Evil King. She couldn't see the Ugly under the Mask and The Snakes were well behaved, steering the car to its destination. She didn't know where they were going but she wasn't frightened.

The car veered and left the busy road. The Evil King and the Little Princess drove down a slight slope and the car came to a surprising stop. The Evil King turned the key and the engine was quiet. They could still hear the cars on the busy road above, *swish, swish, swish* as they hurtled by. The Little Princess and the Evil King remained unseen in their car, down in the dip and there was a sudden silence.

The Little Princess knew she had been Tricked. She knew she was a Stupid Princess. She sat still, and she waited for it to begin. The Little Princess looked down at her lap. She wasn't sure what to do and she saw she had turned into a Little Mouse Princess and that the Evil King had turned into a large cat, and the chase began.

She ran as fast as she could, into the back seat and up the sides of the car. She ran across the closed glass windows and into the driver's seat. She climbed up the steering wheel and scuttled along the dashboard and The Evil Cat flexed his claws and his mouth smiled, but not his Cold Ice Eyes. Sometimes he watched her and sometimes he chased her. Sometimes he pounced with his body landing on hers and other times he calmly stretched out his vicious paw and pinned her down, one claw piercing her skin. No one saw the Little Mouse Princess or The Evil Cat because the cars were too high on the road above. *Swish, swish, swish.*

Thump, thump, thump, went The Little Mouse Princess's heart, but she didn't make a noise because no one would hear her anyway. She looked out of the window and wished she had turned into a bird in the sky, not a Mouse, but she hadn't. She was a Stupid, Weak and Useless creature.

The rotten stench returned, and The Snakes woke up. They curled and twisted around the steering wheel, the gearstick, the seats and the floor and the ceiling until she could see nothing but vile Snakes and Evil Cat. More and more Snakes came. They crawled through the air vents and kept coming until there were so many in the car that the Little Mouse Princess could no longer see out of the window to the sky and trees above. *Click, click, whirr, click* went the cameras in her mind. A cold, dark Shadow fell over the car. Finally, there was no room for the Little Mouse Princess and her whole Body was invaded by these rotting, Evil creatures. They writhed and probed and pushed until the Little Mouse Princess was so full of Snake and Cat and whiskers and fur that she could no longer breathe, and she knew she would surely die.

The Little Princess felt her soul slipping away and she cried out in anguish, but she didn't die. The Snakes began to crawl away and there was more space in the car. The Little Princess could breathe again and when she looked out of the windows, she could see the trees and the sky again, and she could hear the *swish, swish, swish* of the cars as The World carried on as if nothing had happened.

But it did happen! cried the Old Witch from within.

'Shut up,' the Little Princess replied.

The cameras in her head had taken lots of photographs, but none were clear. They were blurry and full of snakes and the Little Princess didn't want to look at them. The Evil King picked up the Mask from where he had carelessly discarded it, placed it carefully upon his face and began to drive up, out of the dip, and the Little Princess busied herself. She collected every picture in her mind and she filed them in a Black Box. This box she labelled, *The Lay-By*.

She put the Black Box away, with all the others, behind a Big Black Door. She locked and bolted The Door in her mind. Her soul was captured but she reminded herself she could still breathe.

I survived, she said inside her head.

Exploring 'The Lay-by'

To: Sophie
From: Pat
From what you have written here and the questions you asked me, I think what you suspected happened most probably did. Clearly, he stepped up his abuse in the car and for you to feel choked, it was much worse than in previous situations. By this time, he was sure of your silence. More memories may come back after this,

To: Pat
From: Sophie
I can't sleep. I am replaying it in my mind and feel so overwhelmed. I wish I could be stronger now.

To: Sophie
From: Pat
I would suggest that once you have written as much as you can, put it away mentally where you keep your notes. You already remember clearly much of the awful abuse you endured, so ask yourself, how does it help you to go on torturing yourself? More may be revealed in due course. But now you must ask yourself what, if anything, can I do to achieve closure, justice, and shaming him?

Chapter 16

Blood and No Tears

Mermaids have no tears, and therefore they suffer more.
– *The Little Mermaid,* Hans Christian Andersen

The Little Princess sat in a sea of red.

The blood poured from both nostrils and would not stop. It was the middle of the night and the Butterfly Queen fluttered backwards and forwards with tissues and wet face cloths and the Evil King stood nearby, watching.

The Little Princess was calm. She knew there was nothing she could do anyway, so she sat still and surrendered and waited for it to stop as it usually did, but this time was different.

She used up all the tissues and the Butterfly Queen flew off in search of more face cloths and towels, to absorb this neverending stream. The Little Princess waited for her to come back and tried to catch the blood in her hands. *Drip, drip, drip,* it went on, and her small hands weren't big enough for so much blood and it dripped through her fingers and onto the carpet.

The Little Princess put her head back, but the blood flowed down her throat instead and she swallowed and swallowed until her stomach protested violently, and she added red vomit to the red sea.

The Evil King tried pinching her nose, but the Little Princess moved away.

'No!' she said, and the Evil King stepped back in surprise. The Little Princess glared at him. She knew this was because of him. Her little Body was bubbling with fury and rage and now it was finally overflowing.

She breathed in through her nose, drying the blood, and

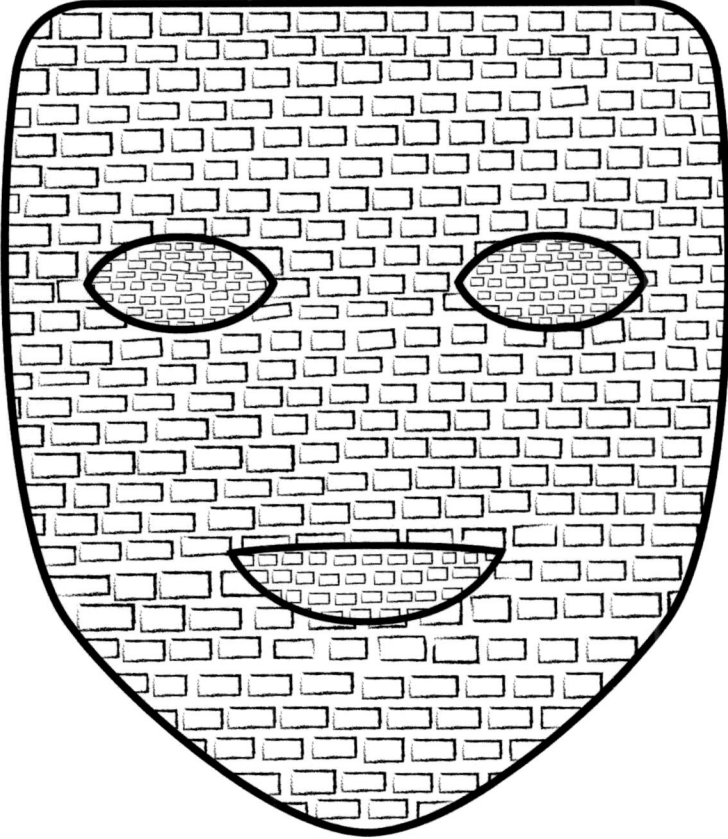

Picture 1 –
'Mask of Bricks'

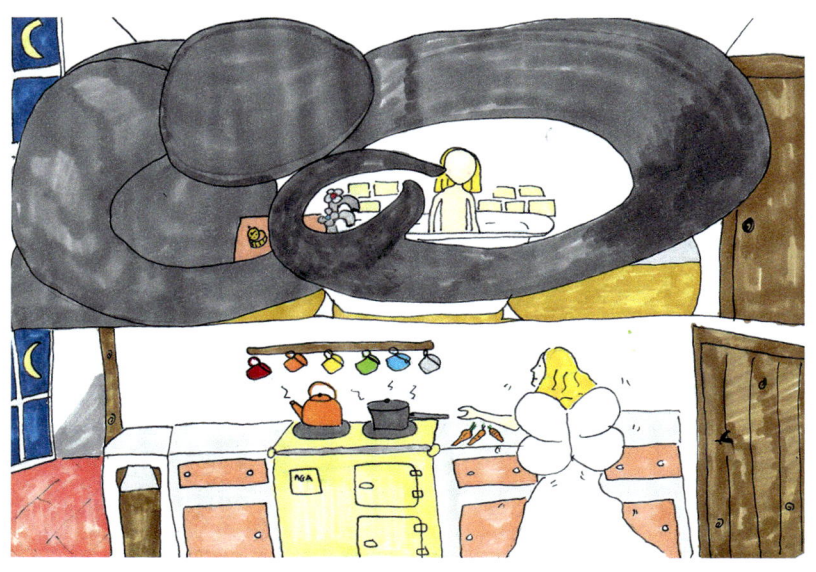

Picture 2 –
'Bath'

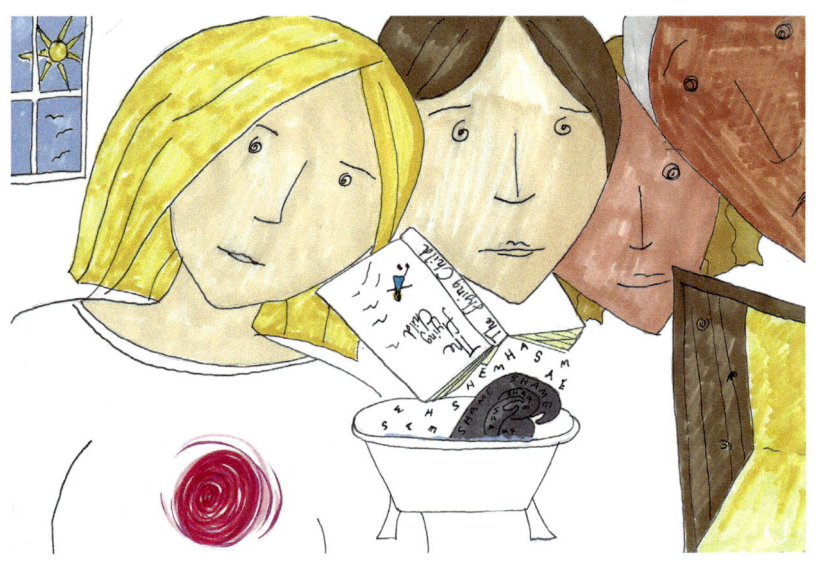

Picture 3 –
'Shame'

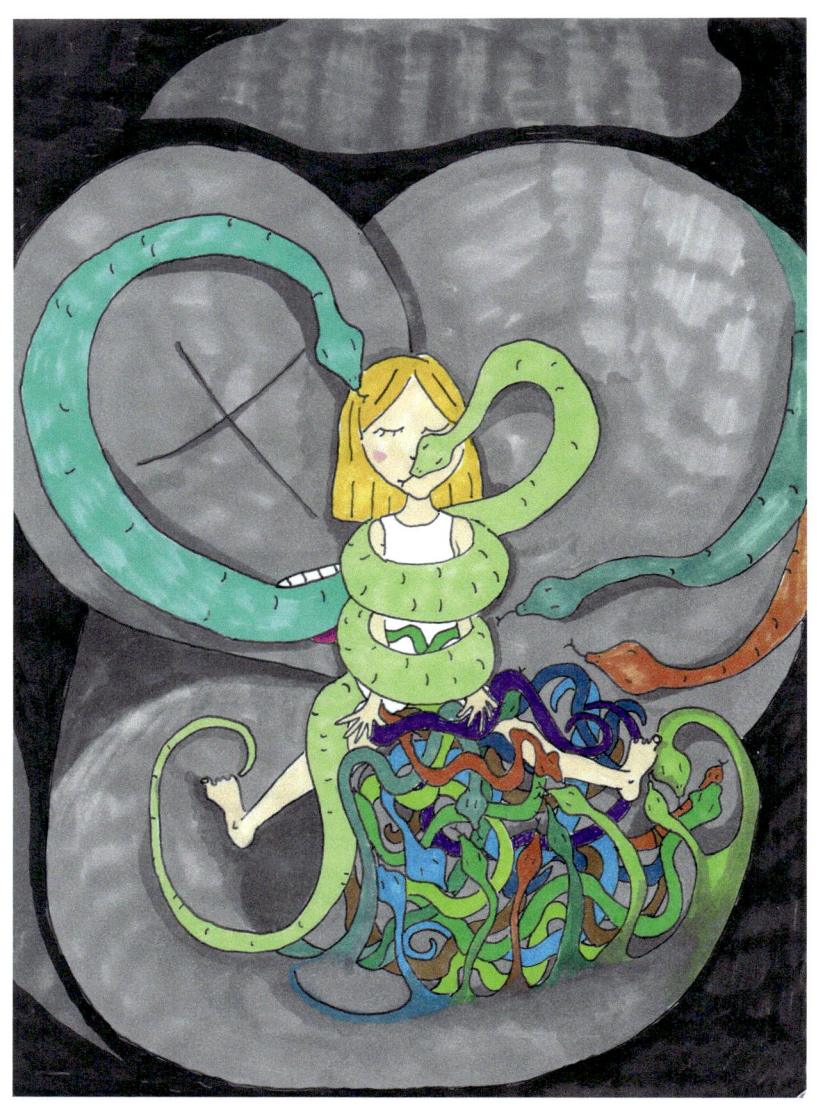

Picture 4 –
'Snakes'

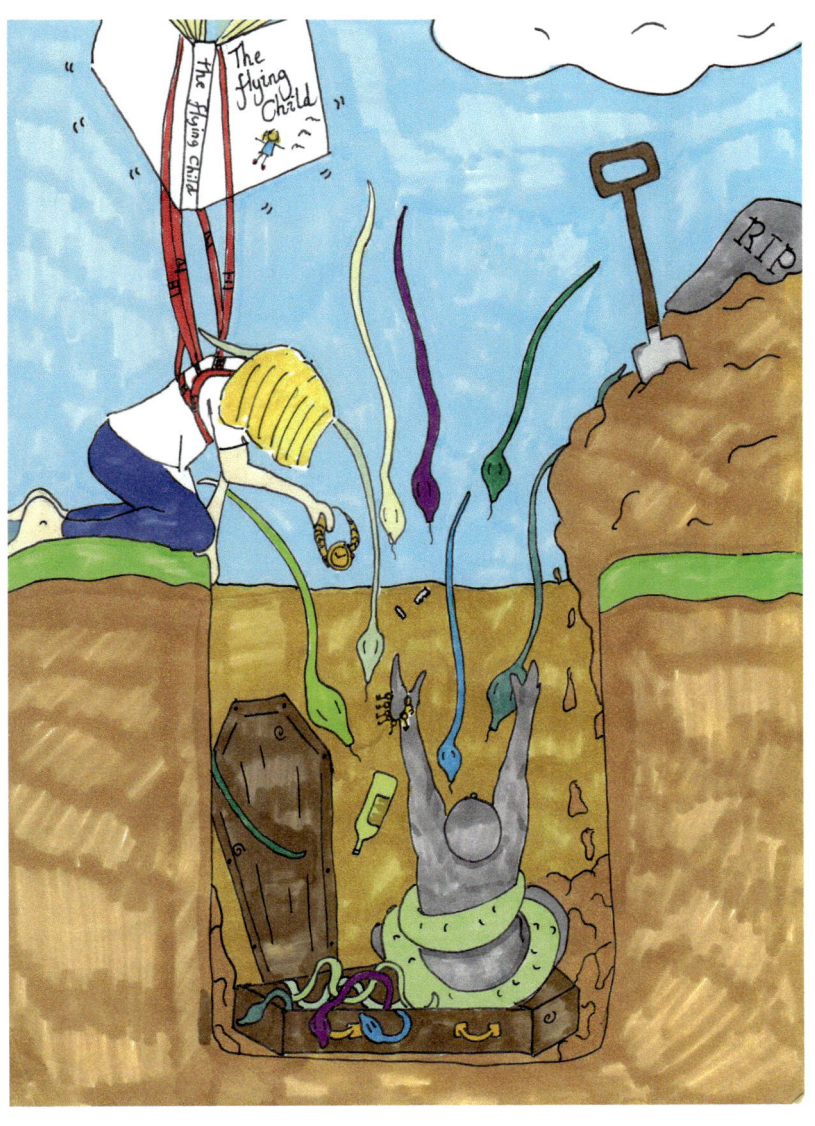

Picture 5 –
'Laying to Rest'

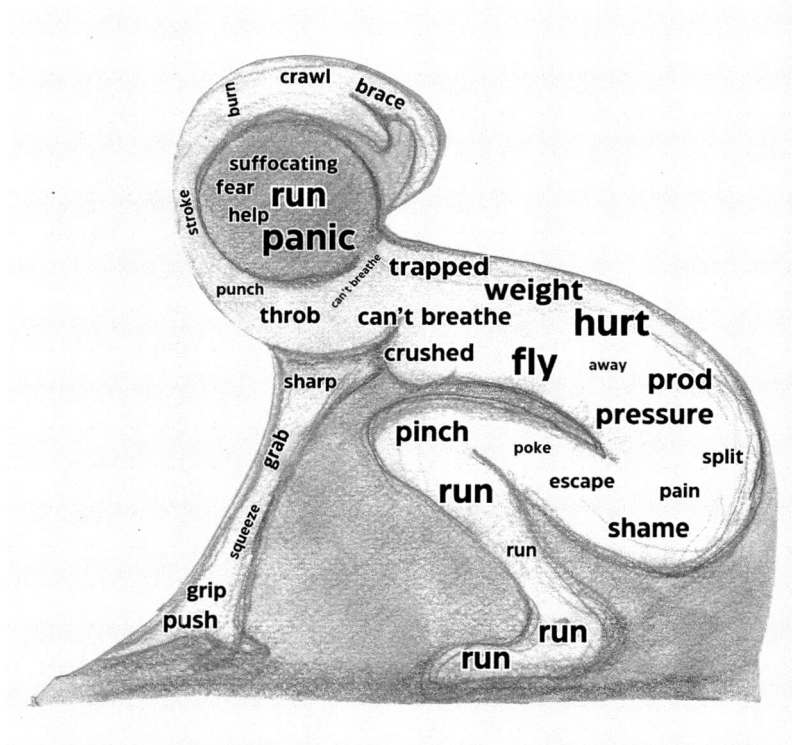

Picture 6 – 'Brace'

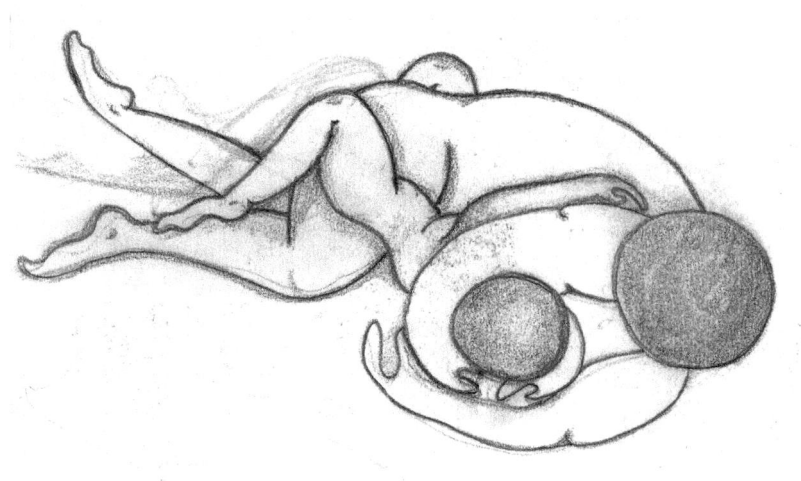

Picture 7

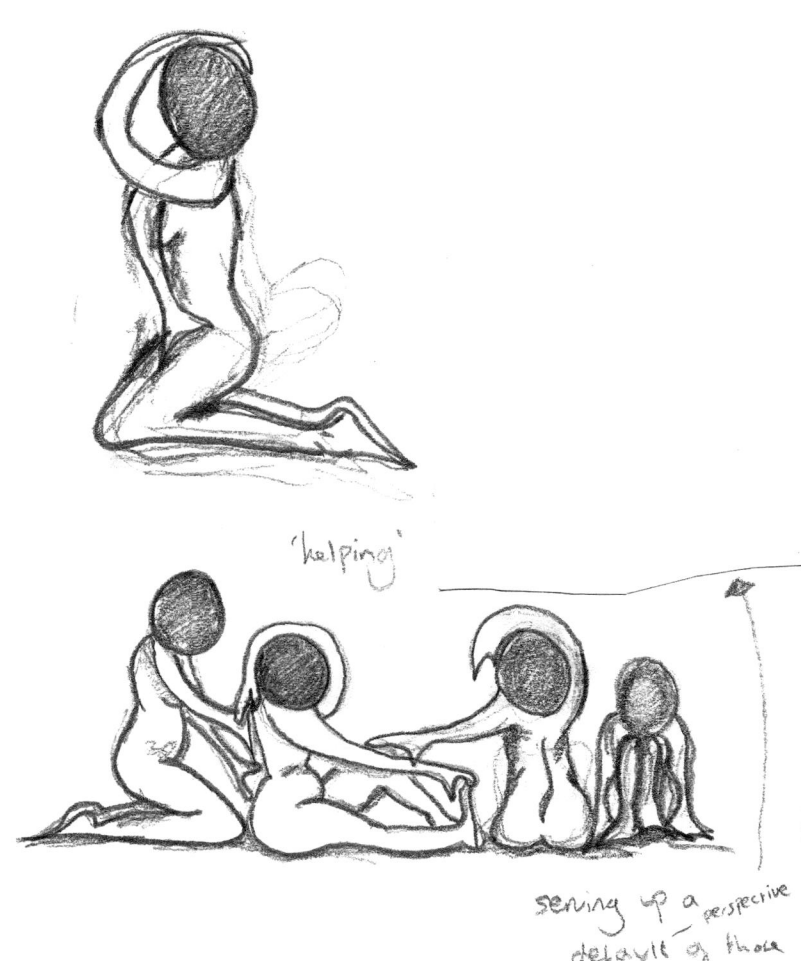

Picture 8 –
'Helping'

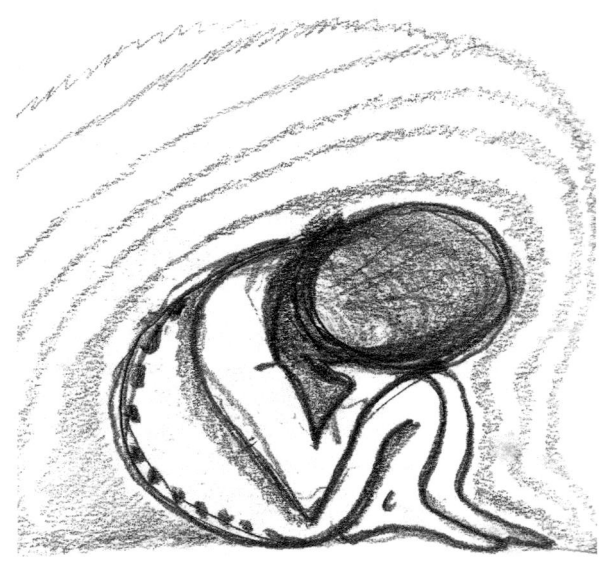

Picture 9

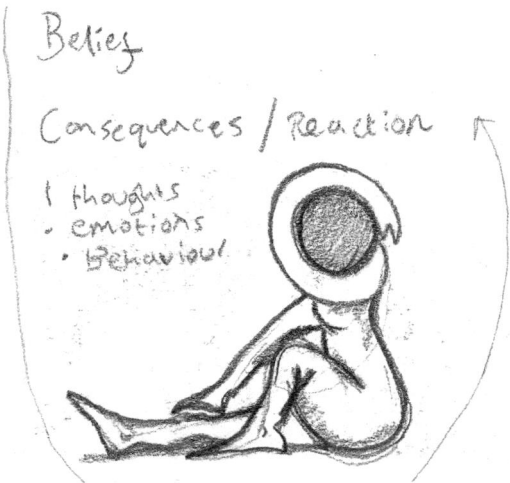

Picture 10 –
'Belief'

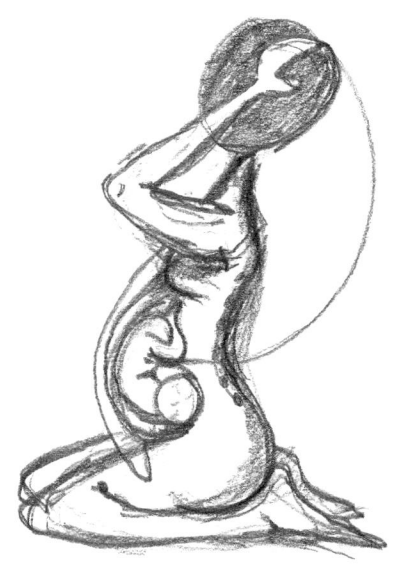

Picture 11

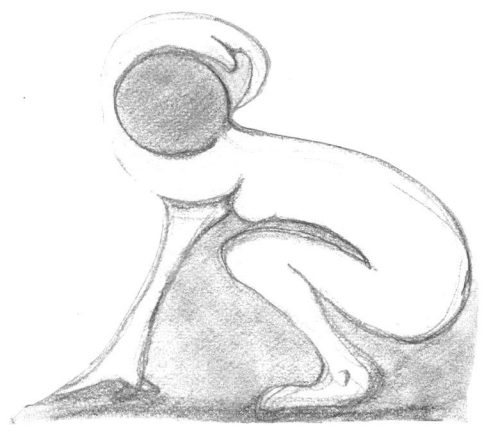

Picture 12

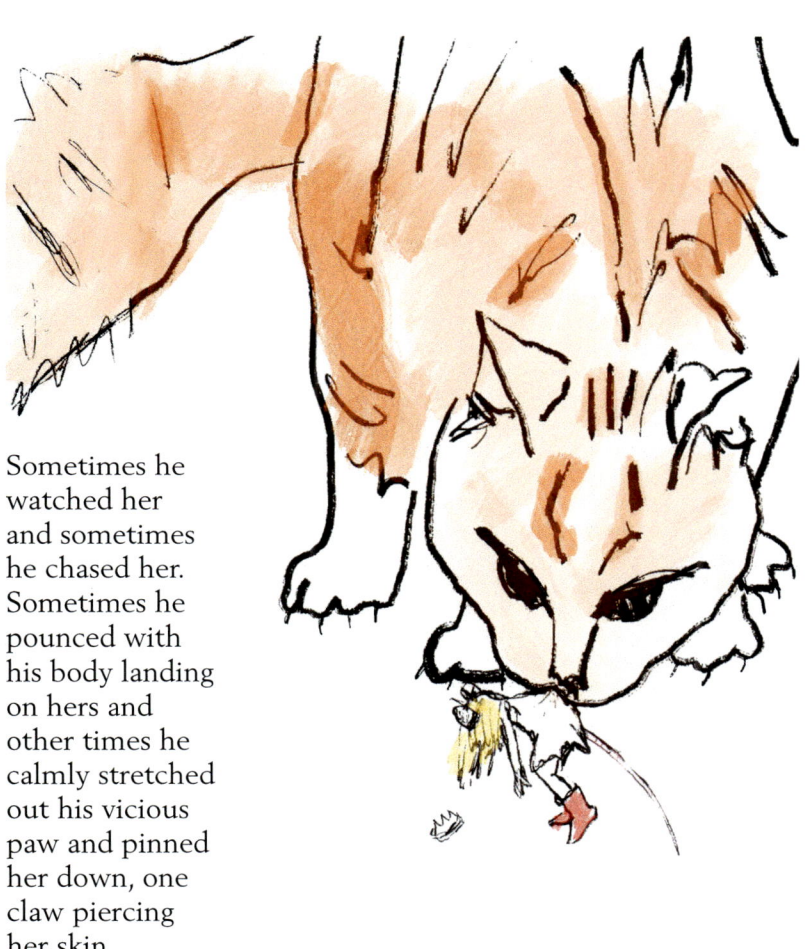

Sometimes he watched her and sometimes he chased her. Sometimes he pounced with his body landing on hers and other times he calmly stretched out his vicious paw and pinned her down, one claw piercing her skin.

Picture 13

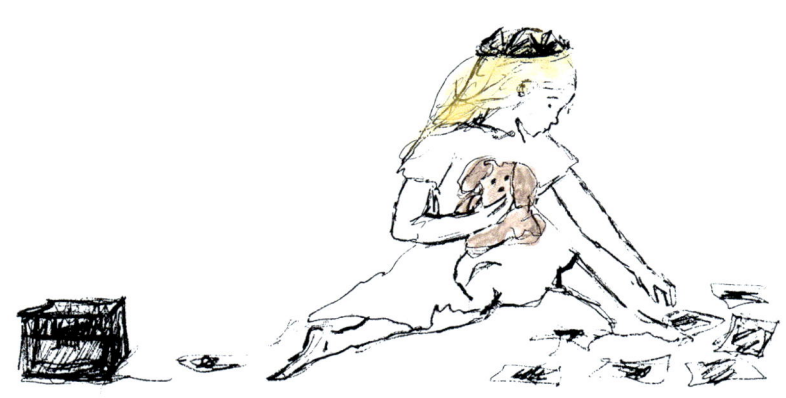

She carefully picked up each photograph, narrowing her eyes to blur images she didn't wish to see, and filed them in a black box.

Picture 14

'What mask do you wear in The World?'
asked the Little Princess.

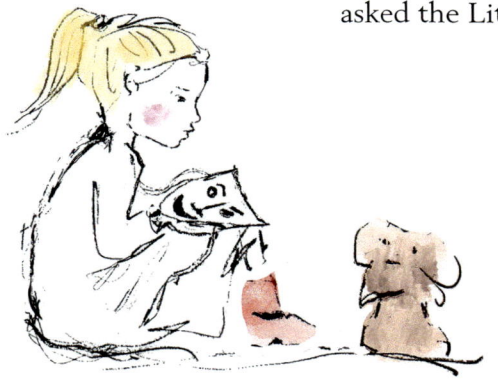

Picture 15

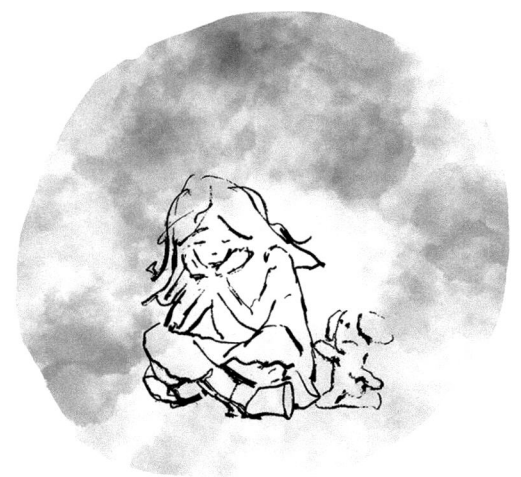

Colour, for the Little Princess, seemed to have disappeared entirely.

Picture 16

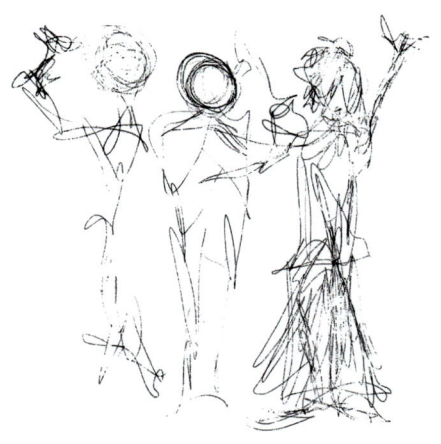

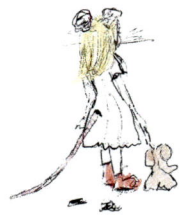

The Little Princess was beginning to think Grown-Ups were quite stupid.

Picture 17

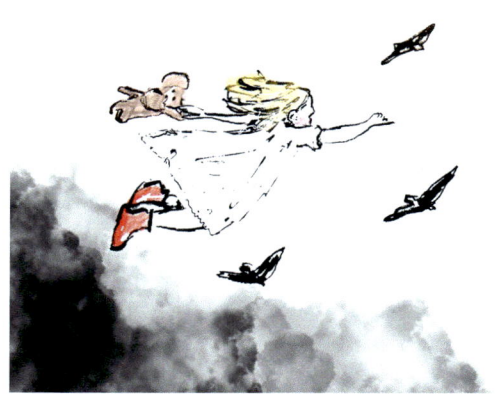

The Little Princess rose from the bed and leaving her Body to the snakes, floated away, away out of the cottage, over the high walls and into The World where the sun shone brightly and the sky was blue.

Picture 18

out through her mouth. *In, dry, out. In, dry, out.* She waited for the blood to clot but there was too much fury and there was nothing at all she could do to stop the bleeding. The *drip, drip* turned into a running flow and the Little Princess's world turned red. Red hands, red knees, red floor, red towels, red Butterfly Queen. The only thing not red was the Evil King.

'We must take her to The Hospital,' he said.

'No,' whispered the Little Princess, with Fear in her heart, and she remembered bright lights and hands on her Body. The Fear made her heart pound and thump and the blood pounded and thumped too, faster and faster it flowed until the Little Princess began to feel so unwell she decided she had no choice but to surrender completely.

Bundled in blankets, with towels wet with blood around her head, the Little Princess was placed in the back of the car, and she resigned herself to her fate.

She resigned herself to being carried into The Hospital. She resigned herself to being placed in a high seat. She watched with detachment as her blood-filled dishes were replaced with new ones.

She resigned herself as she heard The Doctors discuss what to do.

'Isn't she Good?' they said. 'Isn't she calm?'

They couldn't see that she wasn't Good, she was a Frozen Statue, and they poked long burning sticks up her nose and burned away the part of her that was causing all this trouble and still she didn't make a sound. She smelled her Body burning and she felt the pain and still stayed silent. She just waited for it to end.

Chapter 17

The Touch

'I'm sure I'll get along somehow. Everything's going to be alright.'

– Snow White, *Snow White and the Seven Dwarfs* (1937)

The Little Princess lay on her front and the Kind Lady knelt next to her. The Little Princess waited for The Touch. When it came, she was surprised at how gentle and warm it was. She liked the smell of the oil. *Up, down, around and back. Up, down, around and back,* and the hands pressed a little harder. The Little Princess's small Body began to respond to the repetitive movement. It stopped resisting and began to relax. Her arms and legs felt heavy, and the Little Princess began to feel sleepy.

Up, down, around and back, went The Touch. The Kind Lady's fingers touched the Little Princess's neck and firmly pressed and rubbed. The hands continued, *up and down,* and pressed into her shoulders and travelled along her ribs. The Little Princess worried that she would laugh because she was ticklish, but The Touch was firm and determined and the Little Princess closed her eyes and her mind began to wander.

As her muscles softened, so did her mind. The Little Princess found herself looking at the Big Black Door and it softened and relaxed too. It shimmered and shifted, and the Little Princess's Body tensed. She needed to check The Bolts.

Up, down, around and back, went The Touch, and the Little Princess was distracted. She couldn't keep the Big Black Door solid in her mind, and it continued to soften and shift until it began to melt away. The Little Princess didn't want to see the photographs so opened her eyes and tried to focus on the window, but she couldn't. It was behind her. All she could see was the brown wooden leg of the sideboard and the rough pink of the towel she was lying on. She made a noise. A sob.

'It's OK,' said the Kind Lady softly, 'go with it, relax.' And her voice was gentle and soothing, so the Little Princess did go with it, and her Body relaxed, releasing the sadness, pain, hurt and confusion that it held deep inside tissue, muscle and bone.

Up, down, around and back.

She began to feel so sad. She had never felt such sadness. It made her cry, silently at first. The tears slid from her eyes and rolled into her ear that was pressed against the rough pink towel.

'It's normal to feel a release of emotion' said The Kind Lady, 'let's finish for today,' but she looked a bit worried as the Little Princess sat up.

The Little Princess felt a tap had been turned inside her head and her tears continued. She felt herself overflow.

The Butterfly Queen came into the room and was worried too.

'Are you OK?' she asked gently. 'Didn't you like it?'

But the Little Princess couldn't reply. There were rivers of tears on her small Body. Her hair was wet, and her chest heaved with painful sobs. She felt the tears on her feet, and they ran between her toes.

The Little Princess watched and felt bad for The Kind Lady, who tried to explain to the Butterfly Queen, but still the tears fell.

She cried and cried until her mother put her to bed and still, she cried until, exhausted, she couldn't cry anymore. As she fell into a deep sleep, the Little Princess wondered if she had run out of tears entirely.

Exploring 'The Touch'

I have read your emails and will reply to them later. That was the best trauma release therapy you have had to date . . . that is noteworthy. You are growing something completely awesome here.
She must have wondered at the copious number of tears a young child was releasing. Massage and similar holistic therapies do that as they touch the emotional centres. She was skilled to bring such a result. I often found when I practiced reiki that by the end, the client would be pouring tears. That signals release.

You don't do massage, do you? I would trust you.

No I don't, but it sounded as though it did you a power of good.

There was a quote on the radio that is fitting for my book. It was a programme about Frieda Kahlo.
'When something so personal is represented so truthfully, it becomes something universal.'

That's beautiful.

Am I Attracting Darkness?

Would you ever use a Ouija board?

No, I don't like them . . . too dark.

I agree. He did. I wonder if something happened, and it made him what he is today.

Dark people will attract dark things. Why would you want to contact entities that could have potentially awful effects on you . . . too awful.

I think he was a teenager.
But I worry that I'm doing the same now.

That's the worst age to play these games. I understand your fears, but your aim is to help others and you are not doing anything to him at the moment.

What if he senses it?
Reading that back I can see how irrational it sounds.

You need to gradually detach from him, without anger, hatred, or malice, and then he will no longer have a hold on you. He feasts on making others dark.

Yes, but I'm risking making him interact with me again on some level.

You have to think how he connects with you, if you don't do anything.

What do you mean?

You feel helpless and mentally unwell.

Yes.

So, you don't deserve to live like this.

It is something I need to do, to move forward. I need to find courage. I also need advice on how to protect myself from whatever angle his attack could come from. [that could take any form] if I push him too far and he flips. Guns are a part of my story that I haven't really touched upon.
But I also recognise that the fear could be a result of a very clever, calculated psychological assault and that it was nothing but smoke and mirrors.

* * *

Well, I started to write, wrote the word, 'guns', then decided to move a couple of glasses from my bedside table, to take them downstairs. Dropped the glass. It exploded on the wooden floor, and I have shards of glass in my lower legs, feet and hands. Honestly, you couldn't make this stuff up. It's like a horror movie. I'm really cut. Blood everywhere, glass in my feet. If that isn't a sign, then I don't know what is.
You may think I'm crazy but please let me know if you're home safe tonight. I need to know that this darkness isn't drawn to you too. Nutcase Sophie.

Hi Sophie, yes, I am home safe tonight and I'm so sorry to hear what happened. Have you seen to your legs and covered them properly to make sure they don't get infected?

Thanks. They are not bad. Looked a lot worse than it is.

It must have unsettled you when that happened and you are not a 'nutcase'. You ought to be out of it completely given what you have gone through.

I think you've seen me out of it completely at times and so you are just being kind.

I'm writing about guns, and I keep running into a dead end. I'm stuck and can't get past it.

The guns chapter is maybe too 'explosive' to look at right now.

Am I Attracting Darkness?

> I may be totally wrong, but I've often thought that the sexual bit wasn't even the point. Maybe you'll think that that's a strange thing to say but it's a feeling.

No, it's not strange and go with the feeling. The sexual abuse for any abuser is the ultimate invasive control of another. It is not about the sex but about what it does to a victim. That is why it is used as a weapon of war.

> I think there are levels of it too. Not that it makes any difference to the impact on the person being abused sexually but I think there are some people who have poor impulse control who may recognise it's wrong, then you have the people who put themselves into sections of communities where opportunities are more frequent to act upon their depraved urges. Then you get situations like rape in war.
> Then you get the Fred Wests, Jimmy Saviles, Ian Bradys. Something quite different I think entirely.
> No worse for the victim, unless you're murdered obviously. But in terms of the sexual bit. That's how I think of [the perpetrator]. Like them.

Later that night.

> My anger is coming back. I'm so fucking angry. How do I stop myself turning it against my own body?

Go for a walk. Anger is part of recovery and you have a lot to be angry about. Think what you will do to deal with this monster, but DON'T DESTROY YOU.

> This isn't about him.

What is it about?

> I've fucking failed again and I'm bleeding. I'm angry with myself. So, I want to hurt even more. What the fuck is wrong with me?

Is it worth harming yourself for? Deep down the anger is about him, because your coping mechanisms would have been different, and you wouldn't have suffered the way you have.

No, it's not worth harming myself for. But it's too late.

Find some way to expel the anger. Are you going to contact [the psychiatrist]?

No. I'm not unwell. I just need to leave.

OK, then make sure you go back home.

What a bloody awful mess.
I can't stop cutting. Why can't I stop? I'm going to end up in hospital or dead.

Because you are so angry and don't have another way to cope right now. I think you should ask [the psychiatrist] about this because it is happening almost daily and is now getting dangerous.

I feel embarrassed to have let you in on this. I never talk about it with anyone really.
I have an appointment but it's not for another week.

That's OK, it's better someone knows about it as it is getting more difficult for you to control.

They can't help me with it. They will suggest therapy, which I'm doing.

Do you want a call later?

Are you going to tell me you can't help me anymore?

Why would I do that!

Feels like it's all getting a bit heavy.

So, would you like a chat at your usual time, or would you prefer to wait until Monday?

I can wait for Monday.

**To: Pat
From: Sophie
Subject: Guns**
Dear Pat,
I can only get this far.
It may all be a facade and I hope it is, but I have lived in fear of him killing me for as long as I can remember. I don't think he'd care much if he was caught, and I don't think he'd be too afraid to do it. But it's all just feeling. I don't know why he had the guns at all.

Chapter 18

Exploring

> 'Since you have been into that room,' he cried, 'against my will, you shall now go there against your own. Your life is ended.'
>
> – *The Forbidden Room*, The Brothers Grimm.

The Little Princess lived in a cottage, in the Kingdom named His, separate from the rest of the World.

When the Evil King was there, his shadow enveloped the house and gardens and the Little Princess would shiver with cold and rub at the goosebumps on her arms.

Sometimes, the Evil King tucked up his forked tail and drove away. She knew that he went on an airplane that flew to far away places.

When he was away, she was safe to explore the Kingdom of His.

She explored the sheds, with the workbench and tools and flicked curiously through a Big Black Book that sat under a bare lightbulb in the middle shed, the one that belonged, most definitely, to him.

She soon became bored with this. The Little Princess did not understand the long words in the Big Black Book so she moved on to exploring the large brown wardrobe where the Evil King kept the fine clothes he wore on his trips into town. It sat solidly at the end of a dark downstairs hallway leading to a place in the cottage – a second, more formal, sitting room, kept especially for Christmas.

The Little Princess opened the door and ran her small fingers over the soft suits with shiny buttons, the crisp, white shirts with pointy collars, and she touched the mirrored shoes that sat neatly in a row on the floor of the wardrobe. She saw a shelf at the top but couldn't reach it, so she dragged a chair from the sitting room, climbed up and explored. Her hand closed upon a bulky object, wrapped in fabric.

It was heavy and she nearly fell off the chair in the effort of lifting it down from the high shelf.

She wondered what it would be and was surprised when she unwrapped the cream-coloured cloth. It was made of gold. *Treasure!* thought the Little Princess and her hands closed around the barrel and she put her small fingers through the trigger.

'Bang, bang!' she whispered. Her voice was loud in the hush of the house as she was alone. The Butterfly Queen was fluttering in the garden and the Big Princess was hidden away in her bedroom.

The silence rang in her ears and the Little Princess felt afraid but she didn't know what of.

Quickly wrapping up the gold gun she climbed back on to the chair and hastily pushed it back onto the high self.

Shutting the wardrobe door as quietly as she could, the Little Princess dragged the chair back into the sitting room and ran away, out of the dark, cold hallway and into the light of the garden.

Exploring 'Exploring'

To: Sophie
From: Pat
I get chills when I read this and given his complete disregard for animal life, this would naturally extend to human life. I feel we are getting close to understanding the ultimate fear, which is, will I be killed today, and if not, then when? That is why you are 'stuck' with the guns because they were the most terrifying of all. Allow yourself to rest regarding this one. If info comes then write it . . . if not, then let it be.

To: Pat
From: Sophie
This one is so hard to write. The others come in one go but this doesn't.

To: Sophie
From: Pat
This feels very scary and unfinished . . . do you remember what happened next?

To: Pat
From: Sophie
Yes, some of what happened next, I remember, but there is one part which isn't clear. It's terrifying. It's not like the other memories and doesn't have clarity so I'm not sure. I think that is what stops me from writing more.

To: Sophie
From: Pat
OK, you have struggled with the guns all along which makes me feel that it's one of those memories which have been deeply suppressed like the lay-by, because it is too traumatic to process. It is not wise to go any further than the unconscious will allow you to go. You are aware that the memory is there and for the moment that is enough. It would probably be terrifying for the adult you are right now . . . for the child it must have been deeply terrifying.

Chapter 19

Another day, when the Evil King was back in The Kingdom of His, he summoned her to his hallway.

The Little Princess ran, her bare feet slapping on the cold stone floor, from the light of the sunny outside into the icy chill of the dark hallway. She stopped abruptly when she saw the Evil King. He stood by the open wardrobe. The cream cloth-wrapped object was his big hand.

The Little Princess's heart jumped and thumped in her chest.

Grumble grumble, said the Old Witch.

'I see you've been exploring,' he said.

The Little Princess looked down at the floor.

'I'm sorry' she whispered and waited, but to her surprise, the Evil King laughed.

It was a sound that the Little Princess didn't like to hear. It sounded like a laugh, yet it didn't feel like a laugh. Laughter was lightweight and happy and infectious, it bubbled and bumped and made others laugh too.

The Evil King's laugh was flat and empty. It wasn't full of bubbles, it was hollow, and when it reached The Little Princess, it fell to the floor. It didn't make her laugh. It made her want to hide.

'Would you like to see more of these?' asked the Evil King and he unwrapped the golden gun.

The Little Princess didn't want to. She wanted this day to end.

'OK,' she said and walked slowly towards The Wardrobe.

She shivered in her summer dress and stood in her bare

feet and watched as the Evil King lifted down another cloth-wrapped object. He handed it to the Little Princess.

'Unwrap it,' he said.

The Little Princess unwrapped it.

It was heavy and black and looked like guns she saw on the television.

'Hold it,' said the Evil King quietly.

The Little Princess glanced at him and saw the Cold Ice Eyes looking back at her. She started to shrink, and the gun grew heavier and heavier until she was worried she would drop it.

The Little Princess held the heavy, black gun with both hands and the cloth fell to the floor.

He showed her how to open the gun and she saw the glints of gold.

'Bullets,' he said.

He told her that if there was a gap, it wouldn't fire the bullet.

'Try it,' he said.

The Little Princess wondered what it would feel like to die.

Exploring
'Exploring (Part 2)'

To: Pat
From: Sophie
This is as far as I can go.

To: Sophie
From: Pat
That's fine, Sophie . . . no need to go any further . . . The fear factor is chilling enough . . . What you describe is close to the sort of feeling you might get in a round of Russian roulette. There is really no way to describe this monster is there? It never fails to amaze me how you are able to write this story and not be in long-term psychiatric care, and the fact that your story has been incarcerated for so long.

To: Pat
From: Sophie
I'm not exactly sane though, am I? A sane person wouldn't do what I've done to myself. It was healing yesterday but today it's the same as before, soaking through my sleeve.

To: Sophie
From: Pat
What you have done to yourself is a deeply ingrained coping mechanism which goes back into very early childhood and is a trauma response which I personally would not call madness. I am concerned that this is still weeping and the long-term effects if it is not treated. It would be useful to have your wound looked at to get advice on what treatment it needs. Of course, it is entirely your choice. If you are insistent that you will not see GP or go to A&E, it would be prudent for you to understand why it is not healing.

To: Pat
From: Sophie
Do you think one day I will look back on this and say to you, 'Do you remember when . . .?' and I will not be able to imagine being like that again?

To: Sophie
From: Pat
Yes, I do think you will look back on this one day and know that this type of coping is over. It will no longer be who you are. You are not mute, broken little Sophie anymore, but a woman who has found a very powerful voice and as this grows stronger, when she is having a wobbly day, she can ask for help. She will know how to be kind to herself and how to comfort herself like she does for her own children. Shame and guilt will have been taken by the birds to a faraway land.

To: Pat
From: Sophie
I hope so. I really do.

Chapter 20

Three years later, the Little Princess was playing in the garden when she heard the phone ring. She carried on with her game. She was practising running in bare feet on the small, hard pieces of gravel, without stopping. She was good at this game and could hardly feel the stones anymore.

She stopped as the Butterfly Queen came back out into the garden. The Little Princess saw her face and knew that something was wrong.

She crept up unseen and listened to the Butterfly Queen who was talking to her friend. The voices were Anxious and rushed. Some words floated away before they reached her ears, but others were terrifyingly clear.

'What choice do I have?'
'He said he's going to kill himself.'
'He's got his shotgun.'
'I've got to try and talk to him.'
'What if he comes here?'
'What about you?'

The Little Princess shouted in fear as she saw the Butterfly Queen fetching her car keys and she grabbed at her wrists and arms, trying to pull her back and keep her safe.

'Please don't go!' she screamed, but the Butterfly Queen didn't listen. She got in her car, and she drove away to her death. The Little Princess thought that she'd never see her again and her fear turned to hatred.

I hate you. I hate you, raged the Little Princess inside her head and her heart. She couldn't believe that this was how it would end. The Butterfly Queen had chosen the Evil King over her and now she was never coming back, and she hated her for that.

Defeated, she felt her heart freeze to ice.

'Good,' said the Little Princess, who didn't want to love anymore.

Gathering

I am unable to recall much of the session that led to me writing the next chapter, *Summertime* and I wonder if I dissociated – something that still happens to me at times of stress. I do however recall the surprise of seeing my watch and jewellery on my lap at the end of the session. One of the vivid body memories involved my wrist being gripped and I had unconsciously removed my watch and bracelets whilst exploring these memories with Pat. I continued to process this difficult event after the session in messages.

> **Last night I sent you an email and, like before with some of the others, I now feel very uncomfortable about what I've written. Please can you tell me if you have read it and if not, maybe don't read it yet?**
>
> I read it late last night, so I didn't reply then. I'm not sure why you feel more uncomfortable about this one than any other things you have told me. I suspect it is because it is similar to the car episode.
>
> **I don't know either. But I do.**
>
> It may be that it's another confirmation of what you know, but are not yet ready to process.
>
> **I think it's that the memory retrieval is different for the sexual abuse, apart from the bath and some bedtime occasions, and the time when he came back when I was ten and abused me when [family members] were in the other side of the house. Which I haven't written about yet.**
> **I've sent you the rest of the chapter. I've also amended a bit from another chapter.**

To: Pat
From: Sophie
I have been writing this since this afternoon. It's a race against time when I start as I fall asleep. I can't get any further.

Chapter 21

Summertime

'Farewell, farewell,' said the swallow, with a heavy heart, as he left the warm countries to fly back into Denmark. There he had a nest over the window of a house in which dwelt the writer of fairy tales. The swallow sang 'tweet, tweet,' and from his song came the whole story.

– *Thumbelina*, Hans Christian Andersen

The Little Princess woke up.

It was summertime and her window was open. The air was new, and the Little Princess felt new too and wide awake, as she stepped out of bed.

Every morning was the same. After the Evil King left for The Office, the Little Princess would look for the Butterfly Queen. Barefoot, her little feet would pad along the green carpet, down the long and narrow corridor, leading to the Butterfly Queen's bedroom.

The Little Princess stood at the door. It was slightly ajar. She could hear sounds from downstairs and she wondered if she was too late and if the sounds were of breakfast. She pushed open the door and stood on the threshold.

She stood still for a moment, looking at the shape in the bed and trying to make sense of it. Black hair instead of blonde. Large instead of small. Blue eyes instead of brown. The Evil King instead of the Butterfly Queen.

The Little Princess froze. She stepped back. One hand on the door.

'Good morning,' said the Evil King. 'Have you come to give me a cuddle?'

'Stay Back,' the Little Princess heard the Old Witch whisper inside her head, and she knew the noises from downstairs were made by the Butterfly Queen and that she was far, far away – along the corridor, down the stairs, through a shut door, through a room that led to a room that led to the kitchen that led to her.

'Come on,' said the Evil King, raising the side of the duvet, 'come and give me a cuddle.'

So the Little Princess, with her little blonde head and her little bare feet, walked slowly forwards in her white nightdress, towards the bed.

She heard the Old Witch again. *Grumble, grumble*, she went. *Stay back. Go back. Stupid.*

But the Little Princess carried on because she didn't know how to say no and anyway, she wanted a cuddle, and so she climbed into the bed.

The cuddle was brief, and her face was scratched by the scratchy hairs, and she found herself on her back. She was looking at the window. The Little Princess was hot and scratchy too. Her nightdress was now a hard, solid lump, pressing into her back like a clenched fist and her bare legs and stomach shook even though the air was warm. The Shadows were back, and the room was dark. The Little Princess could see the bright sunshine through the window, and she could hear the little birds.

'Fly away,' they said. 'Come out, get out.'

There was a roaring in her ears and a thumping in her chest and she hated the Old Witch, who wouldn't shut up.

The Snakes were back too. Huge and hard and soft, with biting mouths and flicking tongues and they were all over the Little Princess. One Snake pushed and pushed and prodded at her little Body and it pushed the Princess's Body up and up the bed until the top of her small blonde head was touching the wall. The Little Princess cried out as the hard-soft Snake punched her Body and she didn't understand why she was hurting when she'd just been safe and warm in her own bed.

The Little Princess didn't like the lump of hard nightdress pressing against her back like a fist and she didn't like the pushing of the hard-soft Snake, so she decided to go.

The sound of birdsong filled her head and the sunlight at

the window hurt her eyes and the smell of the new air hung in a bubble above the bed. So, her ears left with the birdsong, and she let her eyes be blinded by the light at the window and was glad of it. She didn't want to see. She had to leave her Body to The Snakes and as the rotting, dark and putrid smells floated around her Weak and Useless rag doll self, she rose, up towards the new, fresh morning air. Higher, higher, away, until she wasn't there anymore at all. She became the birds and the air and the sun.

Exploring 'Summertime'

To: Sophie
From: Pat
Subject: Re: Summertime
Good . . . well done, you have finished it and come again to your own realisation and conclusion as why you have [different recall] of the event. The psychologists/psychiatrists will call this 'dissociation'. . . My interpretation is an out of body experience. It is dissociation but more profound than that. There is the 'choice' to not come back . . . potentially to die because you do not want to experience the physical trauma of what he was doing nor the psychological understanding that this [perpetrator] was so immensely cruel and violating. It is the ultimate protection for mind and body, to 'leave.'

> I've sent you another email.
> The body memories have been coming and going today and I have just remembered something quite clearly and it's bothering me a lot because it's a new memory. I don't get those very often as most of the things were never forgotten.

Do you want to email it or not? I can read it later as I'm just about to travel home now.

> It is small stuff but pretty horrid. It tells me more I suppose. I remember the feel of [a part of his body] I thought it was his wrist at first but that it wasn't quite right. I remember feeling confused. I think this was in the dark and that it's a very early memory.

OK, this memory has pieced now with the chapter you read with me, so the full horror of what he did has finally been released by your memory. Now it can be slowly dealt with by your mind.

> I think it's a different time of day though. That chapter was daytime.

I remember [this part of him] was wet, like a mouth or a tongue. The snake analogy with the tongues and bites came from this most likely. Again, this was probably in the dark as I haven't got visual memory, just touch. Sorry. It's horrible to read this stuff. I'm worrying about you and feel guilty sending it on.

At the moment which episode it goes with is not important, it is the fact that you have processed this memory, so you now know it was more than his hands. Do not worry about me. My work is to help take people through this horror to another place.

That shocked me reading that reply, even though I just sent those messages. How mad is that? Even when it's staring me in the face, I find a way to hide from it.

Of course, you will be shocked by what you are reading. It is the one memory you did not want to reveal. You have been struggling with it since it all happened and now you know . . . before you just thought 'perhaps' and squashed it down. You now know the full extent of this monster. Don't try to do too much today, just be gentle with yourself. Now is a time of very deep healing for you and a time to start to live. You are amazing to be alive – I feel I want to send you a hug.

Hug gratefully received.
When I was describing how I felt when I thought I saw him on the street, you asked what I was so afraid of. It is such a visceral fear, like a pure animal instinct. I've always felt it and it is death.

Because you thought all along when you were young that you would die. Every time we leave our body, that is the ultimate choice and for the child it is easier to leave than for the adult.
'Detachment' is going between the two worlds.

I'm losing chunks of time again. Ten minutes or so disappear. It can feel quite frightening, Pat.

OK, shake down, ground yourself with the exercises and do

a task which requires focus . . . some crochet . . . some solid cleaning . . . dishes in the kitchen and say to yourself . . . I have uncovered the worst fear . . . I have always imagined. . . . I have lived through it all . . . and now I WILL BE HEARD and so will others. I am done with the monster.

I hate myself for not being strong enough again, but I hurt myself quite badly last night. I feel that what I'm doing with my story is vital to me moving forward and I'm beginning to see changes already with regards to the power it has but I also feel very vulnerable in terms of my mental health and am not sure of the best way to manage that. Now I have to manage the self-loathing and regret when I look at what I have done to myself. I'm totally putting myself on the line here. I have never been as open about self-harm as I am with you, ever. Not even with myself. I train myself to deal with it and then not look at it again until it's acceptable. Sometimes that takes months and months. I still won't look at one place from nearly a year ago as the cuts were so deep and wide that they didn't heal properly. Can I trust you?

You have trusted me so far, Sophie, and I will never do anything which will jeopardise your recovery. It is not you that you should be giving loathing and regret to. If a young child of 6 or 7 told you this story, would you tell them to go away and loathe yourself and harm yourself because you are to blame? Now the way to recovery is to love that inner child as much as you love your little dog who is with you now and the one who was with you back then. I want you to think about loathing one of your children. You couldn't . . . so why then is that little child inside any different. I would like you to start working with her, with love. When you are quiet and still, go inside and ask her what she needs most and quietly get the answer. That is what I meant about releasing things too fast. You have enough information for the moment. Now it is time to do the most important work. Reach the little child and comfort her.

**This is how it happened. I want to explain it as best I can.
I start to feel emotion – upset or anger to [an event unfolding out of my control such as an argument].
I don't know what to do.**

Panic. This grows.
Self-loathing because I can't stop this. I feel impotent and useless.
Panic grows and I have the physical symptoms of this. Pounding heart, agitation. I want to leave, just walk away and I can't because I'm not even dressed.
I feel like I have forgotten how to breathe and like my head will explode.
I grab whatever blade is nearest and cut. I don't think about it, I just do it. Just once but really hard.
And then I breathe again. I feel my heart rate slowing and I focus on this, but I also have such fear. What have I done? But the main thing is, it stopped my panic. I feel numb to it. I'm breathing again. I go back upstairs, I'm competent, in control, able to [function] in a better way. Hurting myself stops the pain I feel inside.

I'm sorry for so many messages and that I keep jumping from one thing to another and that there's an email thread too. My mind is racing at a million miles an hour and I need to say it unless it flies off again and I forget. That's why I'm not sleeping as my thoughts are racing.

Thank you for these messages and I will go through them bit by bit. Today I am on a deadline for a piece of work I have been doing over the weekend.

I really appreciate it. I feel very exposed and find it hard to trust you with it and only when I get your feedback do I relax again. So, thank you. Am I sending you too much?

No, just keep sending and I will go through it in between my work schedule.

Can you keep track of it?
I'm worried if I send too much that some will get lost and they're all as important to me.

I will work through it, bit by bit, and there are some things I am keeping for our session which is easier to talk through face to face than write about.

Chapter 22

A Little While After

'You are mine, and I am yours, and no one in the world can alter that.'

– The Twelve Huntsmen, The Brothers Grimm

The Little Princess was drawing. In the sitting room, there was a low, tiled windowsill. On the left-hand side, the Big Princess's pile of colouring books and paper sat tidily. The Little Princess's pile on the opposite side was more haphazardly stacked, as she was a more haphazard type of Princess.

She stood at the windowsill and faced the window, absorbed in her picture. She had drawn a green tree, a yellow sun, and she started to colour the sky.

Back and forth went her little left hand. *Cack-handed*, she thought, remembering what The Teachers called her at school. She clutched the pen firmly and started to feel something. The Butterfly Queen had told them the Evil King had gone. He had Walked Out. He had Left Them.

The World was lighter, and the Shadow was gone. The house was quiet and there were no Snakes or Cold Ice Eyes, yet the Little Princess started to feel something she didn't like.

She had a heavy stone in her stomach, and it made her scratchy and cross. She threw the pen back into the box and screwed up her drawing of sun and trees and sky.

'Stupid picture,' she said.

She grabbed a clean, white piece of paper and selected a black pen.

She began to draw. First, she drew the Evil King. Then she drew his new girlfriend, the one he lived with now.

The Butterfly Queen fluttered by and she stopped to watch.
'What are you drawing?' she asked her daughter.
'the Evil King,' said the Little Princess.
'Who's that?' asked the Butterfly Queen, pointing to the other person on the page.
'Sally,' said the Little Princess.
The Little Princess waited until the Butterfly Queen fluttered away and carefully added more to her drawing. First, she drew their faces. Angry, slanted eyebrows and downturned mouths, ears, hair, noses. Then, firstly checking over her shoulder to see she was alone, she added hairs to his chest and breasts to hers. Big round circles, with two smaller circles in the centre.
Then she drew a penis. And she drew a vagina, and she added hairs.
And then, very deliberately, she chose a red pen and began to scribble. She scribbled over their faces and then their horrible Ugly bodies and then, last of all, she scribbled and stabbed out his penis and her vagina and breasts and nipples over and over again, until the paper ripped, and the Little Princess stopped feeling anything at all.
Next, she labelled them carefully, writing his first name above the Evil King's head. *Sally*, she wrote next to that.
The Butterfly Queen fluttered back into the room and the Little Princess was afraid she would get in trouble for her drawing, but the Butterfly Queen just laughed.
'Let's call him You Know Who,' she said, 'and let's call her Silly Sally,' and she laughed.
The Little Princess could see that her drawing had made her the Butterfly Queen happy, but the little girl wanted to shake and slap her, and scream and shout and she was frightened. Now the Evil King didn't have a name at all and how can you speak about someone with no name?

Exploring 'A Little While After'

Did your [family] see all the intimate details of the picture?

Yes.

Were [they] shocked? How old were you?

10.

I would have been shocked if my 10-year-old child drew such pictures.

**I imagine that's what led them to the questions, and to find me the male counsellor.
I still don't see myself as a child. It's just me. If it was my own children, or anyone else then of course, but it's just me.**

Three members of my family and one counsellor asked, separately and on different occasions if I was being abused, but they didn't say it quite like that. I remember them stumbling over words, how they stuttered, used vague language – they were visibly awkward, uncomfortable, and uneasy, and this made me feel awkward, uncomfortable, and uneasy, and I said no. When I saw the relief on their faces, I knew that was the right answer. They never asked me again. Much to my initial relief.

There are many reasons why a child will stay silent, even when asked directly, but all I know is that I replayed the scenarios in my head as a child, and later as an adult. I imagined myself saying 'yes' at the age of ten, rather than twenty years later, at the point of crisis.

I don't hold them responsible because I view this clumsy approach as a result of this culture of silence. As a society, we don't know how to ask these questions, how to speak the words and we need to do better. We are failing our youngest and most vulnerable because of our own discomfort.

Chapter 23

Campervan and Saxophone

'Princess, youngest princess! Open the door for me!'
— *The Frog Prince*, Brothers Grimm

One day, when the Little Princess was playing in the garden of the Kingdom of His, she saw the Evil King appear at the gates. The Little Princess froze. The Shadow passed in front of the sun and the sky went dark.

The Evil King had been away for days and weeks and months and the Little Princess had thought she would never see him again, and now she wasn't sure what to do.

She wanted the Butterfly Queen.

'Come here,' said the Evil King in a kind voice. 'Come and see me.' the Little Princess could see he was wearing his Kind and Gentle Mask. 'Come on! It's me! Come and give me a kiss!' the Little Princess couldn't move. She was a Frozen Statue and she couldn't move forwards or backwards.

Her heart was jumping and pounding with Fear and she could feel the beat in her legs and her toes and her fingers.

She watched as he lifted the latch and pushed the gate forward, slipping inside the Kingdom and her Body felt weighted with heavy stones.

When she knew she would die from fright and waited for the death that was inevitable, she heard the Butterfly Queen and the Big Princess walking up the path behind her. Her frozen Body began to thaw, enough to use her legs again, and she ran, stumbling towards the Butterfly Queen and the Big Princess.

The Butterfly Queen took hold of the Little Princess's hand, and the Little Princess held it tightly.

'What do you want?' the Butterfly Queen asked the Evil King, and the Little Princess held her breath.

'I've only come to see the girls,' said the Evil King sadly and the Little Princess dared to glance at his Mask. She could see the tear in his eye, but she could also see the Ugly behind it. There was no fooling her anymore. No more Tricks.

The Little Princess waited. She waited for him to leave.

'Do you want to see him?' the Butterfly Queen asked her daughters and the Princesses looked at one another. The Little Princess let go of her mother's hand. She understood the Butterfly Queen couldn't help her at all and that she had no choice and for the Evil King to leave again she would have to do as she was told.

'OK,' said the Little Princess,

'I don't mind,' said the Big Princess and they all began to walk with the Evil King towards the cottage.

'I'll see them alone,' said the Evil King to the Butterfly Queen. 'You leave, and I'll see them alone.'

And the Butterfly Queen faltered and started to flutter away.

'Mummy,' whispered the Little Princess and she longed for and hated the Butterfly Queen in that instant.

Her legs were shaking and her head was hurting, and she was so frightened she thought she would collapse in fright, but she didn't. She carried on walking, and the Princesses followed the Evil King into the room used only for Christmas, far, far away from the Butterfly Queen.

The Evil King sat heavily on the cream sofa and told the Princesses to sit with him. The Big Princess perched on the arm of the sofa and the Little Princess sat next to the Evil King.

She could hear the whistle as he breathed air out of his nose. She could feel the heat from his body as it pressed against her, and she was surprised by how big and male he was in her house now full of women. The size of his wrists, black hairs on large forearms and thick sausage fingers. He smelled of Man; musky, dangerous and animal, and of Ugly. She could smell his soap and cologne, but he couldn't entirely wash away the Ugly.

'So, tell me,' the Evil King began, and he questioned the

Big Princess, firing one question after another. What had she done at school? Which tests had she done? What were the results?

He found fault in everything and chastised her. 'Well, that's not good enough. Why did you do that? I expect better,' until the Big Princess looked so fed up the Little Princess feared she may leave too.

She waited and held her breath.

Her turn.

'So, what have you been up to?' he asked, and his tone was kinder, softer than it had been when speaking to the Big Princess. So the Little Princess took a quick breath and clenched her fists and told him about School and her animals, and carefully avoided telling him about their new freedom, without Him in The Kingdom, about the music they played, and dancing in the kitchen, and the Butterfly Queen's friends coming to stay and singing together and dancing and playing instruments.

'I've been playing my flute,' she said quietly, and then very quickly regretted it as she saw how she'd said the wrong thing and that something terrible was about to happen.

'Ah, that reminds me,' he said. 'My saxophone. Where is it? I've come to pick it up.'

And the Little Princess looked at the floor. She didn't dare look at the Big Princess.

Two hundred and fifty pounds, two hundred and fifty pounds, she chanted in her head and feared he would hear it.

'Well?' said the Evil King. 'Where is it?'

The Little Princess didn't know what to do.

She waited.

He waited.

And then, 'the Butterfly Queen sold it,' said the Big Princess defiantly. 'We didn't have any money and we needed to eat.'

The Little Princess glanced at the Big Princess and saw the resentment in her face and she glanced at the Evil King and saw anger and fury in his. She remembered Hard Wood Hands and hurt, and she got ready to run but she couldn't. The Evil King gripped her little wrist, and she began to shrink, smaller and smaller and he grew larger and larger until he was a black cloud of fury and terror in the room. The Little Princess looked at the

Big Princess and could see the Fear reflected in her face and the Big Princess backed out of the room.

'I'll get her,' she whispered, and she left and all the Little Princess could do, like all she had ever done, was wait until the Evil King decided what next. She held her breath and shut her eyes and waited and waited until . . . nothing. She was back to her normal size, sitting on the sofa, next to the Evil King, who was a normal size too and no longer a huge and powerful black cloud.

She wasn't stupid. She was bigger now and she could see his Mask where it lay discarded, in pieces by their feet.

She waited, for the next bit.

Hurry up! whispered the Old Witch from within and the Little Princess strained to hear the Butterfly Queen's footsteps as she came to rescue her. Instead, through the large inglenook fireplace that backed on to the large walk-in larder, she could hear the Butterfly Queen as she fluttered about, feeding the dogs. The Evil King could hear it too and he got up and quietly closed the door.

The Little Princess, sitting on the sofa, had never felt so alone. She didn't understand why the Big Princess wasn't getting help and she didn't understand why the Butterfly Queen had left her alone in the first place and she didn't understand why neither of them were coming back, so she hardened her heart even more and it began to crack and break and weigh down her little Body.

And she waited.

The Evil King sat next to her, and he began to cry. The Little Princess didn't care. She knew it would be a Trick but as the crying continued, she looked at his face and was surprised to see real tears. The tiniest fragment of her heart was still soft and loyal and loving, and this little fragment jolted in sympathy as she had never seen the Evil King cry real tears before.

'Don't cry', she said, reaching for him, and he pulled her onto his lap and held her tightly with his arms as he continued to cry.

The Little Princess felt ridiculous and stupid. She was far too big to be on his lap and she didn't really fit and now she knew what was going to happen next and she knew the Butterfly Queen wasn't coming back and she knew she was alone with the Evil King. She looked at the closed door and behind, at a small cabinet. She studied the ornaments on the cabinet carefully as the Evil King continued to cry. She didn't feel frightened anymore as his fingers slid underneath her clothes, she felt calm, and it didn't really hurt. She couldn't leave her Body this time because she had to be vigilant and listen out for the Butterfly Queen and the Big Princess, in case they saw what was happening.

She didn't want them to see this.

His thick sausage fingers pushed, and she listened to him breathe. It was familiar and she continued to study the ornaments and she continued to listen out.

She never once looked but she felt it all, as he touched her in a place that felt bad, painful, shameful and disgusting all at once, but she still wasn't frightened. She felt Dead.

'I have a new car,' he said when he had finished with her Body. 'I'd love you to see it. It was my birthday last week and none of you remembered and I was all alone.' He sniffed and the Little Princess felt the soreness where The Snakes had pushed and rubbed. The Fear pressed against the edges of her mind.

'I have a birthday cake in my car – it's a Campervan! We can get inside and have a birthday tea party, just you and me.'

And the Little Princess felt the Fear flood back and her Body started to shake and shake. She hated the Big Princess for leaving her and not getting help and she didn't know what to do or what to say. She saw she would have no choice. She knew she would have to climb into the Campervan and she knew that there would be no cake and she knew that the Evil King would drive her far, far away from The Kingdom, the Butterfly Queen, the Big Princess, her dog and her toys and she knew her life would be filled with abuse, although she didn't yet know the word for it.

'OK,' she said, and followed him out of the door, where they saw the Butterfly Queen flutter towards them.

Processing and Writing

At one point in the therapy, Pat and I met outside. I found walking together in the sunshine helped me to speak more openly. I didn't feel under pressure to make eye contact – as I told her more, I heard the birds singing and could see the sky.

Thank you so much for meeting me today. The place was perfect.
Please can I get your opinion on something?
Are there any chapters that you in your role find useful? Or feel might be useful to others and should be in the book?

It was lovely to meet with you today too and the outdoor space was just what you needed. I feel whatever you have written needs to be said and you never know what may resonate with a person. One day, it will be used by many as a form of expression for their own stories. These chapters helped you to come to terms with all the many awful aspects of him, allowing you to 'see' a full picture of just how awful he was. In my opinion each chapter shows us that he is pure evil.
Many victims abused by a close family member will continue to look for a redeeming factor in the person who abused them, but there is none when it comes to abuse. Still, they continue to look, until they finally realise there is none. I feel all of it is useful, particularly sensory input – smell, touch, etc – because a young child is closer to this than language.

OK, thanks, that's an interesting answer. On the flip side, it's important to me that this isn't titillating for perpetrators. I think one chapter I sent you was graphic and that I may stick with the analogy throughout the book but write the actual words, if I feel I need to, for the work that I continue to do for you.

I agree with what you are saying . . . to express yourself for our work and then edit it so that perpetrators would not find anything titillating for them, but that survivors would completely understand it. It is to act as a catalyst for them to tell their own stories.

The Best You Can Do

Spring

I'm struggling today.

So, your fears about your back [discussed in session], I want you to cross through the ones which are 'supposed' fears at this moment in time. If you still want to focus on your back, take one fear for the immediate most important future and write it down. With today . . . write the fears for the day and then pick out the most important fears you have for this day.

My fear for today is that I am not strong enough and that I will take my own life.

What would happen if you took your own life . . . your family would have to bear this. They may see this in the future as a normal coping mechanism . . . list them all down. Each day you are alive – make it matter rather than ending it. Think about what you can do now about your future work and what needs to be put in place.

I wish I was stronger. My mind is my worst enemy. You said you're surprised that I'm not in a psychiatric ward forever after what happened. This is my reality, Pat, this is me. The real me. This is what I became because of what happened to me. This is my parallel life that I shouldn't be in. I'm strong yet I'm weak. I want to help others, yet I make myself hurt.

By helping others, we help ourselves and overcome our weaknesses.
Also don't go to 'the time in the future' because right now it's an unnecessary fear to put in the mix . . . Live life in the moment for now. In the past, your mind was your saviour.

Did you always work in the field you're in now? Do you mind me asking? Tell me to mind my own business if you don't want me to ask.

No, I didn't always work in this field. I was a trained counsellor doing private work on weekends but my main job was an independent domestic violence advisor working with over 30 high risk cases of abuse where, at any time, the victims could be killed by their partners.

Why did you choose this as a career? Why sexual abuse?

Because I had worked with all sorts of abuse situations before. I had done refuge work and community work. Many abused women in relationships have also been sexually abused by partners and as children. Over the years I have known that this is the most devastating aspect of abuse for women, and I just knew this is the area I would finally specialise in.

So, when you listen to people like me, lamenting the life I'm living now, does it make you feel disappointed? I feel like I don't want to let you down.

I never feel disappointed. I am grateful that you can still lament your life because then there is hope that one day that lamentable life becomes a life full of hope and joy.

And if it doesn't? What if you're wrong about me?
Then I have to accept that that was the best you could do.

"Then I had to accept that was the best you could do" were perhaps the most important words I would ever hear Pat say. It was at this point I realised Pat might be able to guide me out of the dark but, ultimately, I had to save myself.

I need you to know that my sessions with you have been so valuable. When I first came to the group, I felt scared, like a square peg in a round hole. Gradually, with time, I came to understand and accept the path I needed to take. I began to

identify with the other women, and I felt less alone. I really thought I could heal.

Go on believing, Sophie. Once you have come through this, you will come to the other side of fear. The dreams are telling you this. Your dreams are telling you how fearful your life was. The unconscious will play them for you, for you to identify what might be helpful in them. Eventually, those dreams and nightmares will stop as this waking one will. No one has any control over life or when it will end. All we can do is the best we can, with the cards we have been dealt, and you are doing just that.

What do you think of psychiatric medicine and hospitals? Do you think I need to go back in?

Only you and your husband can decide that because I don't know how helpful you found it in the past. Some people would not recover if it weren't for psychiatric help. As for doctors, for acute conditions such as fractures, accidents, correction surgery you could not but accept their interventions. It's long-term chronic conditions and their attitude and behaviour towards complex trauma that I find extremely disappointing.

They kept me alive for 6 months in 2010. There is no doubt at all that I would have died.

So, you must decide if and when you are close to this situation again.

Do You Think I am Strong Enough?

I've done some digging. Had a glass of wine to pluck up the courage to ask my family.
The important thing is that this basement [in the next chapter] DID exist. It was a recording studio and accessed from the high street. My mother can't remember if it was through the dry cleaner or next to it . . . but it was a room. She's thinking it wasn't a basement, but down a couple of steps. The windows were boarded up, which is why I thought it was a basement or a dark room.
She had no idea that he took me there, or why he would have had cause to take me there. But the important bit is that this memory is real. She also remembered his 'jailer's' keys. I didn't even know it existed, but it does/did.
She also said that she thought he acquired this room later on. This makes sense of why this is now being triggered by talking about the time in the bed and the lay-by, at age 9/10, rather than in younger childhood and if he abused me in this room, that's why I'm associating it with pain because his abuse hurt more the older I got. What I'm unsure of is what happened first.
What if, being able to speak these words isn't enough to save the person. What if it's not enough?
I feel I'm at a pivotal moment and that I could go either way. Backwards or forwards. I can say, 'He raped me,' but then what do I do? What comes next? Do you think I'm strong enough to stay out of a hospital? What if saying those words sends me back there?

What happens if you take a deep breath, and you accept what has happened to you and realise that there is now no point in entering a psychiatric hospital. Accept the amazing person that you are. Embrace the force that is within you – that saved your life – and go out into the world and tell it how it was. What happens now that you have the words to say what happened? I am glad your mother told you about the basement and confirmed for you that it was there. This year you have done the most amazing work. Slowly all you amazing people will come together and there will be no stopping you all. We can run away in fear, or we can say, I have nothing left to fear because I can never know a greater fear than what I have already endured. Now I stand here fearless, and you will listen. What have you got to lose?

I don't know what happened last night. I called the police, somehow, in my sleep. FFS.

OK, so did they come out to you?

No. I woke to hear a man's voice asking if I needed the ambulance or police.
It was so embarrassing.

Were you dreaming? Given what we have been dealing with, the SAS might be more appropriate!

I had lots of dreams and a very disturbed night. I can't remember them though – only the one that involved you.

OK, write whatever you have. Probably dreams will be jumbled for a while. Don't fear saying things out loud in your room for a while just so it fully sinks in but remember at this moment in time there is nothing to be done with the past. It's done. Consolidate it and then act with a right heart and mind to bring the truth to where it needs to go.

I am writing and I'm sending it across to you by email. Do you want the dream too?

Yes, send that too.

Did you get them? I remembered one other dream from last night. This is a recurring nightmare I have where someone has hooked their fingers into my vagina like a carcass on a meat hook. There's nothing I can do about it and it's painful in the dream. I'm attached to the person until they decide to let go, which they don't.

Dreams

To: Pat
From: Sophie
Subject: The Dream Last Night
This was later, after I called the police. It's shaken me, doing that. It's like when I used to sleepwalk.

    I met you in London. We are working on something together but when I get there, you're upset, and I can see I've done something wrong. Apparently, I have used a hand gesture that is offensive to the women we are working with. I remember using the gesture but not deliberately to offend, as I was unaware it was a gesture at all, and I had been trying to stretch my arms and throw body memories off me.

    I can't convince you and you are so upset and feel so let down by me that you decide to leave.

    I feel shattered that even you can't understand me and that you don't believe me now.

    I feel totally ashamed of doing this thing that has upset you so much.

    I decide to go home too, and a male refugee keeps insisting on carrying my bags, one of which is a plastic washbasket filled with my things. I let him and he is sad too because he can see the sadness of the situation and the wasted opportunity.

To: Sophie
From: Pat
This dream is for you to interpret really because maybe it is your perception of my expectations. The purpose of my role is not to have expectations but merely to act as a guide.

    With regards to you asking me whether you were strong enough to come through this and what happens if you are not, I simply played Devil's Advocate to ask you what the purpose would be going back, for example, to [the hospital]. If you have unfinished business at the hospital, and need to go, then that is your choice as this is your journey. It is also your choice if you wish, to remain there, just as it is your choice to harm yourself or whatever else you may want to do. You now have a choice over these things because your mind is your mind to do with whatever is appropriate for you to do. You are now the adult, he is no longer the perpetrator, unless you wish to keep him with you and carry him along for however many years that might be. I have just taken you on your journey with the limited skills and abilities I have available to me but ultimately you must be your own magician. Now it is entirely up to you what you want to magic. There are no wasted opportunities because if we 'waste' them it means we were not ready for them at that time.

I hope that helps.

To: Pat
From: Sophie
It was an instinctive thing I do to brush the memory of him off me.

It wasn't to do with your expectations of me either, but it was that I was desperate to communicate with you, but I couldn't do it adequately and you misinterpreted me which made me feel hopeless and sad, because if you did that, what about everyone else?

The not-being-believed part – I have always had the fear I would not be believed. I'm talking to you now, so I guess it makes sense why that comes into my dreams.

I'm seeking reassurance from you, because I need it, having started to speak.

I think it's because I now want to speak the words and that is both empowering but daunting. I want you to understand what I'm saying, and I'm frightened that the words will get stuck. I want to do this repeatedly until I can say them without hesitation and fear.

I have had a thought of how to do this. I would like to send you what I have written and when we meet in person, I would like to read it aloud, with you helping me, if the words get stuck. Like you helped me on Thursday, except you would be prompting me with my own words. This needs to happen at the beginning of the session, so that we can discuss it and the body memories have time to fuck off again before I leave.

Do you think that would work? If so, when?

To: Sophie
From: Pat
Yes, the words need speaking . . . voice louder and stronger until

voice no longer wavers. It is spoken strongly and in truth and you must choose the words.

Monday at the usual early slot is the earliest I can do. If you need a call meanwhile, I can do that too.

With regards to believing you, I wish I didn't have to believe such an awful story of cruelty beyond measure, but sadly I know how full the world is of sadistic monsters.

To: Pat
From: Sophie

I was silent as a child and I grew up, silent about it all. I didn't want to think about it because it was too painful and the body memories too awful.

Then I spoke and I didn't receive the 'right' response. I received silence in return, so I was quiet again.

Then, the same thing happened again, and when I told [member of my family] I could see the inner turmoil. I could see it would be easier for her to say it wasn't true, but even though I could see she wanted to [believe me], she couldn't do that because she knew enough about him, but I was silenced again in case other people who didn't understand my family, and what it was really like to live with someone as manipulative and cruel as [the perpetrator], thought it wasn't true.

The thought of having to explain myself, defend my account of the abuse was exhausting, because I couldn't speak the words and so I was silent instead.

Re-writing 'Summertime'

I have rewritten the chapter called 'Summertime' as the child, with my memories. I've described everything that happened in that room, and I've pieced together the body memory of my wrist and words spoken. It is achieving what I'd hoped for, and I am now ready, and want to speak these words.

OK, do you want to send me that chapter and I will look at it later today. You can begin by allowing yourself to say it out loud if you can. You will need these words when you are talking about your book. So if it helps detach somewhat . . . as if you are delivering a talk about YOUR Book so there is a sense of you but it's not too overwhelming for you.

I keep trying to press send and my courage fails me. I need to send it at a time when I know you have time to read it and let me know. It makes me feel too exposed to just send it into the ether not knowing when you'll get a chance to read it.
I'm sorry I'm making this complicated.
Do you think that there will be an end to this fear? It's ridiculous how fearful I am today. I feel so unsafe and it's because I've 'told' even though I haven't actually sent it yet. It makes me wonder if he threatened me to buy my silence and I've forgotten. I have absolutely nothing to base this on, but the fear of speaking is indescribable. It burns through my body and my stomach and I feel so bloody scared all of the time. I'm SICK of it. I feel like running. So stupid. Do other women feel like this?

Yes, all the time. That is why they also don't say anything. I am sure he would have made sure he silenced you with fear and that he will be banking on this even today. Shame, guilt, and fear are the three top ones. All of them ensure silence.

If he found out, maybe he would kill me, but I've been dead all my life because of what happened.

Someone else is reading it now. I have a friend who works for the Met, and she's asked to read it.
I have lost one friend through sharing this book.

Then that friend isn't likely to be any support or help in this next stage of your life and probably doesn't want to hear and doesn't know what to say. There will be many people like that out there.
How are you now you have written in the first person? This is a massive step forward to say 'I' and to describe exactly what happened. It will help to read it out loud so you can hear your own voice.

I'm sorry if it's too graphic.
I'm OK. Part of me feels relief. Another part visualises my boots sitting in my hallway and my coat hanging on the hook and running away. I also feel shame. Anger. No sadness. That worries me. I feel sad when I see you look sad when you hear me but I'm worried that my heart has hardened too much. I do cry in my sleep sometimes though. It's not like I can't, just that I don't when I feel I should, if that makes sense.

I think every part of you can come back to life again. It isn't too graphic for me in that I am glad you can finally express the horror of what he did. I feel sad for everyone who has gone through abuse and it is easier to shut your heart down, but if you can still cry, then you can feel and if you can feel you can live again. Then he has not possessed you at all. I think he would be shocked if he knew you had revealed this. You have no place for shame or need to run away. You have done an amazing job.

I am a bit worried about sleepwalking again though! Or sleep-phoning . . .
I'd assumed that it had stopped but maybe it's triggered at the moment by feeling fearful and unsafe.

It will settle the more you express what has happened. Sleep walking and talking is another unconscious way to express what is happening. Dreams will also gradually subside as you voice what has happened. Of course, people fear they will fall apart but what they don't realise is that not speaking is a coping mechanism. They may feel very scared of losing that coping mechanism because what then? In your case once you have your voice, you will reach many, many people. Your writing is brilliant, that is your forte, your gift, and your voice. **Thank you.**

Even with childhood abuse, once life becomes completely absorbing and purposeful, it does fade into the background. Of course, it never leaves completely but there comes a time when life is so full and amazing, that it slowly loses its hold and brings a sort of acceptance. Finally the long-sought inner peace arrives, because there is nothing left to process, and the question 'why' concerning him, has no meaning anymore.

Yes, I can see that. I'm not there yet but I have hope that I can be there.

I too have strong hopes for this.

Telling My Story As 'I'

I sent 'Summertime' written from a first-person perspective. I have redacted a large majority of the text and edited the descriptions.

To: Pat
From: Sophie
Subject: Summertime – written in first person
[Removed text]
None of it made sense. I had an idea about the facts of life by this age. I even had a picture book. Not once did I think this was what was happening to me. I never equated these furtive, uncomfortable at best, painful at worst, secret assaults on my body with the cartoon drawings of a mother and a father making love and babies.
[Removed text]
Focusing on something made things like this more bearable. I hated the sounds he made when he abused me, the sounds of his breathing. When he [removed text], I would always focus on the window, or if it was dark, on the sounds of the birds scratching in eaves above my head, or a plastic bath toy.
In my bed, I would focus on the window or if it was dark, a bubble of air under the wallpaper. I would trace it with my fingers and try to smooth it out but never could.
When I was taken by surprise, in a different place, I would seek out something new to focus on. I struggled to focus when I was in the lay-by. I wonder if this was because I kept moving or was moved by [the perpetrator].
His attempts to [removed text] – I had no words or thoughts about this, just that I was in this terrible situation, with white heat, panic and pain and that I felt suffocated by him and I was trapped. I knew I must stay silent because he was [the perpetrator]. It felt like it was my fault, for getting into bed and for [removed text]. It felt frightening, violent, unsafe, and very confusing. [Removed text.] This is why I described this episode to you as attempted rape initially, but the body memories never matched up with 'attempted'. I couldn't say it.

Because of the pain and panic and because I couldn't breathe, I remember that I was desperate to get out and see the window and the next image I have is of looking down at myself and being free from my body, watching from above but of turning away to the window.

I have no memories at all of returning to my body, or what happened afterwards, but my body remembers in its own way.

What was clear was that life tilted on its axis that morning. One moment I had been asleep in my bed, and minutes later, I was assaulted in the worst possible way. I was raped whilst my family was downstairs. Then, I had to hide what had happened to me and life was 'normal' again. Something like this does terrible damage to a person's psyche which is very hard to undo, especially when there is a shroud of secrecy surrounding it and it's in the family home, where a child should feel safe. I never felt truly safe again, and then, it happened again. Even when he left the family home, I was always waiting for him to come back and do it again.

These are terrible memories to have, and they were pushed very deep down but not far enough as they never went away. Writing them begins to free me from them. I have faith that speaking these words will release me from that room and that bed once and for all.

Recalling this always resulted in body memories. Out of control, awful body memories, which I struggle to speak about because I've pushed them away for 32 years.

The worst bit of all was the feeling of when he [removed text]. This is extremely vivid and unpleasant. It felt terrible when it happened and continues to feel terrible in memory. I was completely humiliated and degraded when he did that to me. This particular body memory can remain for hours, sometimes days at a time and I can feel like I will lose my mind because of it. It causes me great distress. Writing it is hard. I feel ashamed because I am describing something that in an adult relationship would [removed text] but I write the words in desperation to be free from it. Sometimes I feel it in my dreams. I visualise cutting this part of me away, to counteract the body memory. Drinking, self-injury, and bulimia have resulted from this distress, as an attempt to escape from the feeling – to force the feeling away.

The feeling like I was being punched and that I was breaking.

The feel of his [removed text] – I can describe exactly how that felt.

Feeling unable to breathe, breathless.

Shaking, particularly my legs.

The feeling of pressure on my wrist, the words, the sound of his voice, are memories that have come back as I've worked on this. The room was bright with light, it was warm, I was wearing summer nightclothes. He left in [removed text] so there is a chance that it was just before **then**.

To: Pat
From: Sophie
I'm torn between thinking I'm glad about what I've done and a wish to take the words back again. I felt like this when I spoke some of my story in the groups, so I'm hoping it will pass, like it did before.

Some time later . . .

I am feeling uneasy.

Are you uneasy about what you have written? You have now identified this story as yours. I want you to think about how it makes you feel and where you feel this emotion. Next time we meet, you can read it out loud to me, so I am actually with you as you make it more real, and I'll be there to support you. Take all of this easy. Don't overburden yourself and remember none of this was your fault. As we have already established, there was nothing you could do and no one you could go to.

I am uneasy with what I have written.

I would expect you to feel uneasy about that because it makes it real. That is why you need to take this slowly and maybe read over what you have written a few times and just get to grips with it gradually until you can tolerate what you have written. I am not using the word comfortable but tolerate.

This is where your retreat idea would work so well. At this point, when we (the women) are maybe more stable. To be somewhere beautiful, and to feel cared for, calm, relaxed, with people that we trust.

I feel the urge to do this with you, whilst safe and warm under a blanket, with a cup of tea and the ability to hold your hand if I needed to. It feels lonely doing any of this when I'm by myself.

Detachment

I've just discovered that I must have detached during a conversation today. It was important and something was discussed that I am unaware of. Totally. I discovered this in a follow up conversation and made a total fool of myself. How is that even possible? I must have been talking?! But not fully present.

You can always just say really sorry I have a lot on my mind and cover it . . . That's why a session on Saturday will be good.

If I don't turn up, chances are I'm in a straight jacket in a psychiatric ward.

No way . . . that is not allowed at this stage . . . You have come too far.

It's a bit scary. Actually, it's really scary. I have experienced this before, but it is quite bad at the moment. Makes me feel like I'm losing my mind.

That's why you should check in tonight, even just to sit and focus. It has been a final huge shock and there is a lot to digest but you are now almost through the dark door to the other side.

Have you seen this before? It feels like a type of aphasia, this inability to speak properly.

Don't try to analyse too much. Just call it shock. Because you are in shock, rather like surviving a tsunami or an earthquake. Just sit with the shock and a cup of hot tea and just allow yourself to recover. The worst is now over.

**I don't understand why I was shocked when I knew what happened. I wrote it.
I'm not that child. I'm still not her. I'm angry and don't want**

her yet. Some survivors talk about connecting and loving the inner child. I'm not there. I can't connect.

It will come. I know you knew what happened, but you could never say it or even write it. Now you have and it is time to slowly process. We have only been working together for such a short period of time and you have come very fast and far with this . . . Slow down . . . Stop and let it sink in and be with it for however long it takes. You may want to let your husband know that you are at a very crucial part of therapy and to just be there for whatever you need. Don't compare yourself with anyone . . . You are you . . . Each person's journey is unique.

I did say to him that I was feeling detached and he asked if it was following the last session with you as he noticed it anyway. I can't tell him what it's about though.

Don't worry, we will work with this tomorrow. Make sure you are well grounded driving down . . . also bring some blankets with you . . . They will be good to cuddle up in when you need to and we will work on body memories. The child may want to draw pictures again at some stage if she hasn't got words for expression. This may even take the form of just colours.

Do you mean draw before or during?

Whatever feels right to you.

Shall I bring paper and pens? Or do you have things there?

I decided to try some drawing at home.

This was interesting. I started to draw, and I found it even harder to connect with my adult body than the child's! So, I drew the body memory in the child's body instead. I'm sending it now in case I bottle out tomorrow.

This is what I hoped would happen. I have pens and paper unless you have favourites to work with.

It all seems so obvious though, doesn't it? Should be so simple to understand and work through but it's not.

This is an excellent piece of work for me to work with. Thank you. Of course, it's not simple and sometimes we need a guide to point out the obvious to us, because we are lost and confused. Once we find the path, we are able to find our way.

I drew him as well in the drawing. I started to recreate the drawing I drew when I was ten years old. In his body, I have coloured in the places that represent danger.

Yes, that's what I'm intuiting. It helps me to understand where to work physically as well as emotionally.

Would you like me to send you that part of the drawing too?

Yes, that would be good.

Let me know if you've got the second picture. I've had to delete that one from my phone because I don't want to look at it. It shouldn't delete off your phone though.

(Sophie sends a drawing of both a front and a back view of her child-self. Her body is wrapped in barbed wire. The parts of her body where she feels body memories are coloured in red. The untouched parts of her body are coloured in blue. Her face is masked and there are heavy weights on the top of her head, and her shoulders. The drawing of the perpetrator is as described in *A Little While After* that she recreates for Pat.)

This was like my childhood drawing and I scribbled over those parts of him.

I have received the second picture. These are very important and gives us the beginnings of a language to speak with. This is like the childhood one ... Who saw it? ... Was this what you tried to show The Butterfly Queen? Look at the state of the poor child.

> No, the child wasn't in the picture. That's just my response to current body memory.
> It was of [the perpetrator] – he was on the left-hand side of the page as I've drawn it today. I drew his wife on the right-hand side. Naked, like him.
> I then scribbled over their genitalia and faces.

Yes, the child is in a sorry state.

> I'm trying to draw more but there is someone everywhere I turn. I'm desperate for somewhere to just be. To sit with this pain, fear, and body memory. I'm not sure how to do this in grabbed moments of time. It's impossible. I end up feeling like I'm going forward, then I hear footsteps, and someone comes into the room or someone calls my name and I have to put my mask back on to hide the way I'm feeling. Not very well.

You have done enough and the rest you can do with me tomorrow in peace and quiet.

> **That's all for today.**

We will see where this goes tomorrow. Tomorrow is consolidation day and body memory settling down day because the body memories have told you what you needed to know. They led you to the fear and now out the other side.
Now the r job is done, and you don't need them anymore.

After the face-to-face session . . .

> I am back. Thank you so much for a powerful and important session. I have left feeling positive about this.

The next day.

> **Can I send you some more?**

Of course. I will be running a group for a couple of hours now,

but I can read on the train home this evening. Keep sending . . .
How are you feeling releasing all of this?

It feels good, cathartic. I am skipping a lot now as it was getting too much and fast forwarding to another part of my life. I'll send you this. I want to carry on with the other bits though.
Is it working on whatsapp or is it too long?

No, it's perfect.

Remembering the Basement

I reread my dreams that I had when I was in hospital.
I had recurring dreams about being [removed text]. In one dream, I found a woman and child on a bed and they had both been injured. In my dream I helped them turn onto their sides, like putting someone into the recovery position.
Rereading these dreams is bringing me images of the basement again and these images are filling my head. I don't have clear memories of being abused in that way so why?

Maybe it has something to do with pictures in that basement and the things that might have been stored there. Just take it easy when nothing more is there. Distract yourself . . . go out if necessary.

All feels very dark and horrible. I want to remember what happened in the basement and the car because it's my body, but it feels like it's getting worse and worse.

Detach from this. The mind doesn't want to remember right now. It isn't necessary to remember every detail of how gross someone can be. It's the difference between watching a horrific movie to the end just so we can say we have seen it all, or getting up halfway through and walking out, saying 'I know enough . . . It's vile and I don't need to know anymore because how will it benefit me.'

I don't know if I agree. Maybe for some but not for me. It has only lost its power over me as I learn to speak it. If it's left, it festers inside me.

Then for the moment let filter through only what the mind can deal with. You can't force mind nor body. If you do, it closes down.

I'm not. This is coming to me. It helped me to send it over to you. Thank you.

To: Sophie
From: Pat
Hi Sophie,
I'm taking time to look at the material you sent. The memories triggered yesterday; we can just acknowledge them until anything more comes to the surface. It may be that it could take some time before anything is revealed to you or, of course, it might not happen,
Now it's important to feel what you said last night in session – which is so positive – that you are actually enjoying being you. This is truly amazing. Let that sink in and keep taking this work forward.

Pat, I've been thinking, and I don't remember what I did on that summer's morning after the first rape. I also don't remember going home after the lay-by or even where we were supposed to be going. I have memories of these events with blanks on either side, apart from the basement where I have clear flashes of things before – like the keys and the street and following him – unlocking the door to this 'basement' and then nothing real enough to hold on to. Just bits and pieces. The overall colours in the room – browns and black and equipment. And this image of a man from behind. And above all else, the terrible fear and feelings about this place.

That's OK ... just let these things ebb and flow. Now you are in a stronger place, you may eventually receive the information.

Last night I woke up with such a jolt. I hadn't been dreaming – or can't remember it if I was – but I woke up with the words going round in my head. 'That's it' and I felt I knew it all. But then it went away.

It will come to you when you are fully ready to accept the extent of what he is capable of.

I don't know why it chooses to come now, when I've just spent

the morning with you but I do remember something that went with my feelings of 'that's it'; a feeling of having an asthma attack – of not being able to breathe. In my dreams I mean.

Well, that's OK. You have liberated that. Breathing was a problem when you were first born. Write it down and let it sit until more comes. Breathing and focusing the breath is the most important part of not only life, but of focusing the mind.

So just sit with this quietly over the coming days and see if anything more is revealed to you. I am about to start an hour-long online workshop now so if I don't reply to anything it's because I'm out of action.

Chapter 24

The Basement

'But the blood always remained, for the key was enchanted.'
— *Blue Beard*, Charles Perrault

The Little Princess was excited. She was in The World with the Evil King and he was taking her to The Office.

They stood on a busy street. People and cars rushed by. She watched as he removed a huge ring of keys from his suit pocket and selected one of the largest gold keys. This one unlocked the front door of The Office.

'To the top,' he said, pointing to the stairs and the Little Princess ran up, up, up – one, two, three flights of stairs. She laughed because there were so many and she waited impatiently at the top for the Evil King to catch up.

The Little Princess watched again as he selected another key. This one was medium sized and it unlocked another door, and the Little Princess hesitated, before following the Evil King into the room.

He showed her where he worked. It was light and bright and the Little Princess saw the coloured pens and huge sheets of paper, and wanted to draw.

'No,' said the Evil King, 'there is no time for drawing. We're going now,' and he led the Little Princess back out of the door. She laughed as she ran down the flights of stairs – one, two, three – because she felt like she was flying.

The Evil King locked the door behind him and the Little Princess turned left, back to the car.

'No, this way,' he said, and he pointed to the right.

The Little Princess thought they must be going into town instead.

She skipped along the pavement and the Evil King walked quickly behind.

Tap, tap, tap, went his mirrored shoes.

The Little Princess thought the sound was like a hammer, hitting a nail.

Tap, tap, tap.

The Little Princess heard him call her name, and she stopped. Looking back, she saw him standing by a door, holding his large set of keys. *Jailer's keys,* thought the Little Princess.

She skipped back and was curious. Did the Evil King have keys for every door in The World? She couldn't understand how he knew which key belonged to which door, but he did. The Evil King selected the smallest key on the ring and unlocked the door. Placing a hand on her back he guided her inside. There was a dark corridor ahead and the Evil King pressed a switch, but the light was still dim. The Little Princess walked down some steps and into the room beyond.

A basement, she thought to herself, looking around the room. She noticed that there weren't any windows and that the room was silent. Gone were the noises from the street above. Gone were the people and gone were the cars.

The Little Princess saw microphones, cables and cameras. Dials, buttons and switches.

'Don't touch,' said the Evil King, and his voice was soft in the still of the room.

The Little Princess felt her body turning into a Frozen Statue. She raised her hands to catch the pieces of the Happy Mask as they cracked and fell, dislodged by the fur and whiskers that appeared on her face. She shivered in the shadows that crept from the darkest corners of the basement, wrapping tightly in a blanket of Cold Ice.

She wanted to leave but she was a mouse and was caught in a trap.

* * *

At the end of that day, the Little Princess sat, surrounded by photographs on her bedroom floor. She was busy. She carefully picked up each photograph, narrowing her eyes to blur images she didn't wish to see, and filed them in a black box. Then, she gathered sounds that were scattered around her and as she picked them up, a few escaped through her fingers.

Tap, tap, tap, she heard and the Little Princess held her breath and closed her eyes. She waited until the sound faded before breathing again and carried on calmly, stacking, filing, storing until the box was full. Then, she sealed it firmly with tape. The Little Princess labelled the box, *The Basement*, and she placed it carefully behind the Big Black Door in her mind. Making sure that the door was locked and bolted securely, she walked slowly downstairs for supper.

Exploring 'The Basement'

To: Sophie
From: Pat
Subject: Re: The Basement
Dear Sophie,
First of all, the basement . . . This is the closest you have come to 'memories' of this event and let's see if anything else emerges. You have no need to feel vulnerable in front of me. We have been on a remarkable journey together. I wish the day would come where I never again have to take people on such journeys, and I can sit back on a beach in the sun, but all we can do is keep 'gnawing' away at this subject until it is heard and acted upon.

Hi Pat, I'm sorry to text you to say that I am not coping very well.

So, the purpose of life is to find joy and happiness and to eradicate what has caused the loss of this in our lives. The laws of the land favour predators, paedophiles, and perpetrators. The only way we can change that is by working together, making the world hear that this is a sick way to live. To take up this challenge, and to be really on board with it, our warriors have to be strong and focused with no thought of weakening.
That's how we get the job done.

And when the joy and happiness go and you can't find it, do you fake it? I spent all my life faking.

No, you think back to where you first found it. Being in nature is a good start . . . being with a dog is another . . . My dog is so daft you can't take life seriously . . . That's why I got her – so as long as you can have a dose of happiness once a day, that's a beginning.

I keep writing a message but then deleting it. I feel a desperate need to talk honestly but feel that you can't understand.

Well, you can give it a try and see. It might be worth sending an honest message before we get into anything more.

Yes, we are still meeting, despite everything, because I'm faking, and will do tomorrow unless I wake up and the blackness has gone away. If it hasn't, I'll still fake. I'm good at it as I have had a lot of practice.

Well, it depends if you want to go on faking it or stop everything and re-evaluate. It's perfectly normal to go back to the black hole and even want to stay there. Often its easier than moving forward into the unknown. Black despair is comfortable when we have normalised it. Happiness is alien. We might not even know what it means when someone asks us to be happy. Yet, if we can make the decision to live, we can always try living and happiness out as a mask first. Then others respond warmly to it and eventually over time it becomes a better mask than despair. The despair mask means we become lonelier and nobody, not even those who care about us, know how to communicate with us anymore. Then we miss the best years of everyone's lives.

What's the point of that? Faking is surely better than that? And hope that things improve. I don't feel comfortable feeling in black despair. Not remotely comfortable. I've felt comfortable being able to do the stuff I've been working on. It's made me excited, powerful, given me hope, sense of achievement, a drive. Why would going back make me comfortable? It doesn't. It is such an awful thing to even contemplate going back that I'd rather die.

So why the blackness then if the future looks so much better with doing something useful?

I don't know. I'm scared of it. Why now? Why can't it leave me alone?

When we go to these places, we forget that we are in charge of it all, not some mysterious other. We control our thoughts . . . we control our mind and our bodies and our spirit, not anyone else.

So, we discipline the mind until it functions in a useful way. When we have a thought, we gather it up and we blow it out through our mouth in a sigh. We let it go. If we don't, the mind becomes a dustbin, full of rubbish that never gets emptied and it will spill over into other people's lives and our home, and we will get to a point where we can no longer be bothered. Disciplining the mind is an art. It generally begins with meditation and stillness. It needs patience. The past is the past and can't be changed . . . Find anything useful as you sort through it and use it . . . The rest you let go. It is like sorting out a heap of old clothes for a jumble sale. By the time you have sorted it, you are probably left with very few useful items. The same is true of the thoughts in the mind. Once you have done that, there is space for clarity.

I agree about it not spilling over. I feel alone right now, but my thoughts and actions are dark and far too gone. I will see another day, as I always have done when I feel like this, but maybe I should believe in God for giving me the chance to live another day when the blackness is encompassing me. It makes me act. Or you'd say that I make me act. Whichever it is, I always seem to carry on, don't I?

Absolutely, because one day you will finally say the words . . . I am grateful for my life . . . Imagine how dark and awful it must be to be [the man who abused you.] . . . He has never known one moment of what it is like to see someone's life blossom . . . to really feel the love and bond of an animal . . . or to care for a child . . . or to hold someone in your arms and feel pure love for another human being.

Here is my honest message to you: I am thinking of suicide again.
If I come for the next session, then you should understand as my counsellor what is going on in my head. You don't agree with it, I see your mindset, I wish I could be the same as you and I do have moments of it, sometimes it lasts for months at a time, and I feel the real me – the person I should have been – but the blackness always catches up with me again and I come back to this. Maybe this will stop happening one day, the further I get into driving what we strive for. I hope so.

I'm sorry that I'm not able to fulfil your expectations and that I slip backwards in this way and I'm sorrier that I can't fulfil my own. Tomorrow I may wake up and put the thoughts of suicide away and not think of them again, but I know they're there as a safety net. I will not allow it, I can't allow myself to die from sadness, over years and years. I will take control of my death.
But tonight, now I'm OK. Tomorrow I'll be fine or able to pretend and if I'm not I'll tell you before I leave.

I have no expectations . . . who am I to have expectations of anyone? It is expectations that spoil friendships and relationships. We just do the best we can trying to be the best human being we can, given every changing moment we live through. I did not always think the way I do. There was a time when death and suicide was always in the background as my friend and companion.

Thank you for your time today. I haven't managed not to have a drink. I'm afraid that my drinking stops only when I make an attempt on my life and that I only make an attempt to take my life when I drink. I'm not even drinking that much but it's the way it makes me feel. It's the only thing that controls physical pain. I don't know how to stop it getting that far again.

The only way to stop it getting that far, is to realise what you are doing WITH YOUR LIFE is more important than drinking or taking your own life. It's called living life in the moment so that each moment matters. Then the future moments take care of themselves. Living life as a drinker does not allow you to appreciate and savour each moment because it fogs everything and eventually each moment becomes about alcohol. Your liver is also responsible for muscle and tendon regrowth and so this will ultimately spoil chances for your back recovery. Drinking is destructive on many levels, mentally and physically.

I know.

So run it by your thinking from time to time . . . it does take time to change the neural pathways . . . I do understand that. Your perception of what alcohol does for you acts like a paradox. You go round and round in the dilemma of whether to drink or not, thinking that drinking has a positive side but really there is no positive. Initially it creates a feeling of euphoria but as you know it's false. You know all of this only too well and you do have the power to deal with it. You have done so in the past and your mood was definitely better when you didn't drink.

Yes . . . I know all of this.
I know you're trying to help. Sorry. That came across badly. I will get back to a better place again, I'm just struggling to see how at the moment. Thank you for your help, and for your time today.

I'm going to try and take control of this again by focusing today on the book.

This is a difficult time of year. Today is the autumn equinox . . . equal day and night.
It is a time of death and change as the leaves turn and everything prepares for winter. It is a time of fathers, brothers, sons, and everything that goes with this emotionally . . . so for some it's a sad time of grief and bereavement. Listen to it and allow yourself to feel it but do not immerse yourself too deeply. Have the thoughts, allow yourself to feel and then let them go. Clear out the old and that which is no longer of use to you. Store in your barn only what is useful for winter and spring. Get rid of the rest. The new year will then bear the fruit.

Can I make an appointment to see you again please?

Processing 'The Basement'

I met with Pat where we focused on the basement. When I got home, we talked some more about this through messaging.

> Let me know you are safely back. You did amazingly well today. I am aware that it was a really tough session to say the least. Your book will be heard . . . one day it will fall into the right hands . . . you will need to be ready when it does.

I'm back safely, thank you for asking.
Yes, it was tough and I feel exhausted. Need to keep going with this. Thank you for today x.

> You have come such a long way from the brick mask . . . it's truly amazing. I would love one day for your life to bring you as much joy as mine does, watching people cut the chains; walk free and take others with them. There will come a day in this part of the world, where every child matters. Xx.

I was thinking about it on the way home. It sounds so awful to say I can't feel joy when I have children of my own. I feel their joy but not my own, or if I do, it's fleeting and not often. I think there is an exception and that is music. I find music makes me feel very deeply.

> Yes, you need to go to the place of sadness and acknowledge it . . . Sadness is part of life. It's important that we find a contrast to sadness, or life becomes depression and that is not living. In circumstances like this where joy is only a fleeting glimpse, finding a purpose is vital. Immerse yourself in that purpose. When you do then the magic begins. I would like you to think about the amazing thing we call 'mind' and to invite you to explore it from every angle. Train it to get beyond fear and there you will find joy and purpose . . . go within for these answers as you have been doing this all your life.

I don't normally feel sadness. I feel depressed or low or nothing or when I drink, angry. Sadness is new and I feel it today.

I feel it more strongly for my mother than for myself. She never wanted any of this to happen and didn't deserve it. She's not a bad person. He did such evil things to us all and left us with this legacy to resolve and damage to undo. I want to put myself back together again.

Sometimes I wonder if karma is working against me. Maybe I did something awful in a past life and this is the consequence. Sometimes I feel tormented. I'll give an example of something that just happened . . .

I'm listening to a random selection of songs on Spotify, and on comes the song that immediately takes me back to being in the car with [the perpetrator] to the lay-by and I sat and listened to it for the first time for years and years. I could feel what he did in my body, and I was unable to turn it off. Why would that happen today? Why now? The playlist I chose was full of quite different songs. The lyrics at the end were so clear and they are 'are we living in a land where sex and horror are the new gods?'

I know that is an impossible question to answer. I don't expect an answer. I hate hearing an internal voice telling me 'what's the point?' and I wish I could shut it/ myself up.

It's terrible how it freezes you in that snapshot in time. Rather than leaving my body now, as I did, being faced with a trigger like that song, I seem to leave my adult body and go straight into my child body and feel maybe more than I did at the time. That seems so cruel, doesn't it? I wonder if other people experience it like that.

Maybe if this is the worst bit or the hardest part of the work I'm doing, that it has to hurt to get better. Right now, I wish I was in a trauma centre or retreat. I wish I wasn't here in my house, surrounded by people I love, who can't understand; people I have to pretend to.

> Sex and horror are the new gods, but no one wins . . . it makes for an awful world.

I can't bear it. It's so strong and vivid. Is it what is described as flashbacks? It makes me want to cut out the bits of me he touched. I tell myself it isn't the same body anymore, that our cells replace every few years, but it doesn't work. I will continue with the exercises when I go to bed tonight. I'm sorry to message you so much tonight. Thank you for your replies and for your time.

Just picking up again, Sophie . . . no worries about messaging. You have had a lot to deal with today. These are flashbacks . . . today you have acknowledged what you always knew deep down may have happened, happened. You voiced it and named it and it is both a release and an acknowledgment of horror. Now there can be no more thoughts of 'maybe it didn't happen'. As this reality sinks in, and the acceptance of what he did also sinks in, then the horror of it can go no further and you will progress to the other side of fear. You cannot cut out what he did to you, nor can you change it. Love of yourself is the only way to heal. He is a dirty evil monster, but that is not you. You are a brave, beautiful human being. The path facing you now is to deal with this stuff in the way only you know how. For this you need to make your body strong with the assistance of the mind. You have the gift of writing and an ability to make contacts, along with the driving force of 'fire'. These are a formidable combination. Go out there and be no longer silent or fearful. You will find a way. One Indian woman changed the law, one UK woman changed the stalking law – and so it will happen. All with the same common goal to make this world a better place.

Is it OK to talk about the flashbacks?

Of course.

I can't talk about the worst ones as I can barely acknowledge them myself, but one is my right wrist. Sometimes when I've worked on things with you like today it feels unbearably restricted by my watch or bracelet and I am left with that sensation today. It feels like I'm being gripped by a hand, though I can't remember being restrained by him, except in the wrist. In the body memory, it's a very strong sensation.

This may well have happened when you were out of body, and you felt it when you returned. The body pain and injuries would remain even if the soul had left, because once you returned you would have been aware. As for the more awful body memories, don't go there at the moment. You have had enough to deal with today.

It doesn't feel injured, just pressure.

So, pressure would probably have come from him. Your body is telling you more of the story.

To: Sophie
From: Pat
Subject: Following on from today
Hi Sophie,

With regards to the basement memory, this is where the body memory, although awful, may well be a useful clue as to what you think happened there. It's important for you to realise the repercussions of childhood abuse. It's not just the coping mechanisms but the extremely dangerous and risky situations you find yourself in.

If I had been walking in your shoes and walking your path, I do not know what I would have done. My job is to listen and to guide you out of this pain, until every last part of the horror has been given its voice, until you can only find compassion for Sophie. Then you will be ready to work with and for others because the compassion you finally feel for yourself will then radiate out to others.

You never asked for all this awful stuff to happen to you, and everyone around you let you down. Your experiences diminished your self-worth and left you feeling, believing and telling yourself that you are 'no good'. Feelings of 'I must be unlovable otherwise why would this be happening to me?' became engrained in your psyche. So, you become the worst and most cruel judge of yourself.

This is probably the most awful aspect of childhood abuse; the self-loathing makes the task of living inside your body and mind almost impossible. That is until you take charge of your mind and give it a complete workout and training. Then the body learns to accept and to change also. Old, harmful coping mechanisms become redundant and self-loathing transforms into an understanding that your body is a part of you, but there's also a bigger part and that is your soul.

Your soul has a life purpose. Once you find this, the life purpose becomes all-consuming and everything else falls away. You become you and you are no longer your abuse, and you are doing something you never thought was possible. The further you stretch your mind, your body responds and there are no longer any intrinsic limitations except the ones you want to place on yourself.

I am glad once again you can see how far you have come. Your only fear now is to truly let go of the past so that it no longer haunts you. Now is the time to work on that fear. Winter is the season for that . . . Then comes spring and fear turns to anger and motivation and then summer comes bringing joy and happiness.

Take care,
Pat

~ Part Four ~

Integration

Becoming Whole

Summer

The Flying Child Project – an integral part of The Flying Child CIC – brings lived experience into the heart of professional settings, and it was sparked by a conversation with Dr Clare Brunet, the headteacher, after a safeguarding session I had been invited to attend as a parent volunteer. I hadn't given much thought beforehand to the meeting and what it might cover, but when the topic moved on to Child Sexual Abuse, I was curious to observe my own reaction. I was encouraged to see I wasn't triggered. My heart didn't pound. My face didn't flush. I didn't feel like the spotlight was on me and that everyone was looking at me because they would *just know*. I didn't feel like running from the room and there wasn't white noise in my head. I was able to just sit and listen . . . and reflect.

After the session I asked to speak privately with Clare. Whilst aware I was OK, I was concerned that if there were other survivors in the room, they may have felt triggered simply by the words Child Sexual Abuse. The session had also left me with the feeling of – *is that it?* I felt as a survivor that so much more could have been said. I wondered what the safeguarding training for staff members was like and how the topic of CSA was covered. I started the conversation with, *I was one of those children. I was sexually abused in my family home* – words never said like this before, unprompted, through choice, and what followed played a significant part in the development of The Flying Child Project.

Clare used what is wonderfully described as 'professional curiosity' and she asked me questions such as, *What was I like at school? Had I disclosed? What barriers did I think stood in the way of disclosure as a child? What would I have needed from staff at that time? What did I think were the signs I showed?* Nobody had ever asked me this before and I walked away from the conversation with the distinct feeling I had given her information she could not have gained from a book, a resource or even professional training from non-survivor 'experts'.

As I drove home, I couldn't stop thinking about all of the other survivors. I was just one, and whilst my experience was important, it wasn't just about me. What about all the others? What about the adult survivors still silent about their abuse? Their stories were equally important and yet professionals working with children were blissfully unaware of them. I began to hatch a plan.

Later I was to go back to Clare and describe my idea of a project to bring these hidden voices into educational settings, to give context to the staff safeguarding training in schools, and she agreed to let me pilot it in her school. I reached out to the survivor community, explaining my idea and asking for anyone wanting their experiences of school considering their own hidden sexual abuse to be brought into the project, in the form of quotes, to please get in touch or fill out a short survey. I knew what indicators I'd shown at school and decided to do my own research, tracking down an old teacher of mine. I wanted to know how these indicators had been perceived by staff.

> **Something amazing has just happened, Pat. I remembered a teacher from school. He was so kind and gentle. A shining light. He responded and he remembered me. He's going to give it some thought and let me know if he remembers anything about my behaviour. I was 9 when I was in his class, which was the time of the most severe abuse, I think.**
> That's incredible you are really pushing this forward in every way you can. It's amazing . . . you should take up detective work when you are finished. How did you track him down?
>
> **Google. Then Facebook and I struck lucky.**
> **I feel quite emotional after messaging him. It was like I put one foot right back in the past.**
>
> You never know whether other members of staff said anything when they were together in the staff room. Nothing happens by coincidence, so clearly even if he acts as an emotional trigger that may be important. Sophie, you have to put all this together as a book. It would help so many people.

I'd like to. I don't know if I can do that though.

You might one day when you can look back on it. It was really bad. I say it again, how you came out of it all with such a beautiful mind, is nothing short of a miracle. It gives one hope through all this darkness.

What do you mean by darkness?

The darkness that these awful things leave behind . . . when children struggle to tell their story as an adult. So many painful memories. It is like seeing a small horse trembling in a stable, where its spirit has been broken. It neither wishes to stay in the stable nor does it wish to come out, as everything has become fearful. Their world has changed forever and will remain so until it can slowly learn to trust again. Building trust allows the light to gradually return.

Can I put those words in my book?!

Yes of course, if you like them.

The message I received from this teacher was both shocking and validating. I had sent a school photograph of myself at the time to jog his memory and he replied, delighted to hear from me but apologetic too. *I'm sorry I didn't see your pain,* he wrote. *I do now, in the picture.* He went on to describe his memory of me as, *someone troubled, nervous and with a cowering demeanour* and then defensively continued with, *but what could I have done? In this day and age, teachers can be seen to have evil intentions if they ask probing questions.* I shared his message with Pat. It troubled me.

That is a very lovely message, and he did 'see' but didn't dare 'speak' about what he could see. It is a new validation for you.

So, he did see my suffering then. He just turned away.

He did see you suffering; he turned away because he didn't know what to do. Discovering abuse in a child or adult is not an easy thing to acknowledge, because how do you draw this information out without scaring the child or adult more. Think of the frightened foal in the stable. How do you get it to even stop trembling?

Then if it's so hard, what is the point in the project? I can't change that.

Yes, you can, because you know what it feels like. You have insight on how to speak to the child and build trust, not just ignore it. Trust is the most important word here. If a child can learn to trust someone, then their spirit begins to return. If not, they remain trembling and awful things continue to happen. Survivors hold the key. As [a member of peer-support group] said, they should have shown a picture to the court of her at the age it happened, so they stopped viewing her as she is now, a middle-aged woman. All this insight and knowledge needs to go to the top decision-makers to bring about change.

But how can you gain trust? I don't know if I have the answers even though I know what it feels like. I have very fond memories of this man and I absolutely trusted him and felt very safe with him.

So, if he had asked some questions, you may have told him?

I don't know. I didn't tell when I was asked by three people on different occasions.

That was family . . . might you have told someone outside the family, and think back to what might have triggered you into saying something if it was asked in the right way.

I don't think I would have had the vocabulary.

But you might have been able to draw a picture or explain through doll play or sand tray play.

Yes.

So, there might be the answer to kids who are voiceless.

> It's the strangest feeling today. I've never had any validation whatsoever and what he said was possibly the closest I'll ever get. I asked my [family member] what I was like at school. [They] said, happy enough, had friends, and did well.
>
> I'm so glad you got in touch because yes, he has validated it. I can't believe they didn't see that. I hated school and was desperately unhappy. I never wanted to go. Maybe I never said as much.

Messaging this teacher proved to be invaluable research for the project, mainly because we could presume that things have come along significantly in regard to safeguarding practice in primary schools since the 1980s. But at the time of writing, this man is still a teacher, albeit a lot older than he was. I wonder what he'd do now if he had the same instincts and I wonder how many times over the years his gut instinct has told him there's something not quite right, and he's said nothing, for fear of how he may be perceived by others?

I recognise the challenges we face. How can teachers be encouraged to listen to, trust and act upon their instincts when as professionals there are things they're told not to do, for example asking the child leading questions? This can feel quite daunting and some, like my teacher, may not ask any questions at all. I liked this teacher, and I trusted him. Had he instigated a conversation with me, I may have felt able to talk about what was happening.

Nothing may have changed if he'd acted upon his instincts but by doing nothing at all, he ensured that nothing changed. What if he had logged these indicators? What if the abuse had been detected? What if I'd been helped to recover at an earlier age? What might my life have looked like instead? Would I have dropped out of my degree, struggled with my mental health? Would my survival strategies have spiralled out of control in quite the same way? Would my body have reacted in the way it did? I don't hold him responsible, but I do believe his response is one of the best examples of the culture of silence around Child Sexual Abuse.

Chapter 25

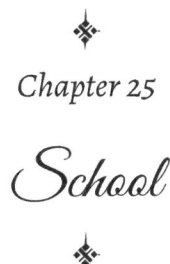

❖

'Cheer up, child. It'll turn out all right in the end. You'll see.'

– Mrs Potts, *Beauty and the Beast* (1991)

The Little Princess left the cottage every day, making sure her Mask was stuck firmly to her face. She didn't much like being at School because she had to keep the Mask on all day. It was hot and suffocating and she found it hard to make herself understood so she decided not to say much at all.

She didn't like to stay in one place and when she wanted to curl up and sit quite alone in the quiet, she couldn't. She didn't like having to listen as it made her tired, with no room to think, and as she sat at her desk, she could feel the bites from the Snakes who had come the night before.

Once, the Little Princess found a hole in her pocket, big enough for a small finger and she rubbed and soothed the soreness away, but she saw her teacher looking, the Little Princess looked away in Shame, trying to hide her hot, engine red face.

The Little Princess felt stuck to her chair and desk and trapped in this place called School. Her little Body was rigid with the worry of being noticed and she thought they couldn't see her if she wasn't there, so she travelled away in her mind. She sat quietly, day after day, wrapping her hair around her fingers and pulling at strands whilst looking through the glass of the closed window and daydreaming herself out of there. No one seemed to notice that she was only half-there at all.

Another day, The Teacher said, 'We shall go swimming.'

The children chattered with joy, but the Little Princess was so frightened at the thought that she didn't know what to do. Her insides violently bubbled and boiled with the worry that she may have to take her knickers off, and in her Fear, she shat in her knickers instead.

The Little Princess bowed her head as the children walked past, holding their noses, and wished that the ground would swallow her far away to Australia, but it didn't.

Her teacher reminded the Little Princess of the Butterfly Queen as she flittered and fluttered but said nothing at all, opened all the windows and put her in a class with the babies. The Little Princess sat in her own mess and waited for the day to end.

One day, the Little Princess cried on her way to school.

'What's wrong?' asked the Butterfly Queen and the Little Princess told her tales of large classrooms and The Teacher who shouted and the too many children who made her head hurt with their noise. The Butterfly Queen told The Teacher and The Teacher put the Little Princess into another class. This one wasn't called Lower, Middle or Upper, it was called Remove and was where The Teachers put the children who couldn't write or read or tie their shoelaces and the Little Princess felt ashamed to be one of them and wished she hadn't said anything at all.

The Little Princess entered the small classroom, and her head was weighed down with her Mask, her Shame and her worries.

'Welcome!' said a kind voice, and the Little Princess looked up.

Another man, warned the Old Witch, but she studied his face and liked what she saw.

He was small and his shoulders were narrow. The Evil King was tall, and his shoulders were broad.

His face was brown, and the Evil King had a white face.

His smile was big, and it reached to his eyes and the Little Princess couldn't see any signs of Cold Ice.

The Little Princess decided to trust him and she sat down at her desk. She liked being in Remove but the worry about being Different weighed heavily upon her soul.

Exploring 'School'

I Was Different

At school I was:
    Quiet and withdrawn.
    I looked out of the window.
    I probably appeared lost in thought.
    I was told to stop daydreaming.
    I would pull my hair .
    I would search for split ends.
    I would suck my hair.
    Nail biter.
    Finger picker.
    Uncomfortable, sore due to the sexual abuse.
    Tried to soothe myself without being seen.
    Frightened of authority.
    Frightened of raised voices.
    Hated to be singled out or asked to read aloud.
    I would agonise over putting up my hand to ask to go to the loo.
    I avoided groups of children.
    I often preferred my own company because I felt different to the other children. I was different.
    I hated PE/games. I hated everything about it. The changing, the energy, the teamwork, because I was never part of that or chosen to be part of that. I hated the humiliation of others during games, not just myself but others, particularly the boys who weren't any good at it, or the ones who were made to take part in their pants and vests because they'd forgotten their PE kit.
    PE teachers were the most unpredictable of all. They sometimes touched the children. A guiding hand on the back during gymnastics, or they would force our necks into a painful position if we couldn't manage a forward roll. They would touch our feet to search for verrucas or run their fingers through our hair during a 'nit check'. They would shout, loudly, all the time and blow deafening whistles that made me jump. Everyone seemed

to shout in games apart from me. I didn't understand the rules of netball or hockey. It always felt so irrelevant, unimportant, and stupid, a waste of time, and I wasn't interested. I never understood why others loved it so much. I hated being cold. Being cold is actually quite a trigger for me still.

The showers afterwards were the worst. From 11 years old onwards we were made to take communal showers. There was a huge room and you had to leave your towel on a bench at one end and walk naked across the room to the open showers, watched by a hateful teacher. I would watch her, looking at the girls' developing bodies and feel rage. When I was 13, something inside me snapped. I went up to her fully clothed and refused to shower. When she started to lose her temper, I called her a pervert and she recoiled. I expected to be sent to the headteacher, but she never bothered me again. She could never look me in the eye after that and it made me feel powerful.

Even after my abuser had left the family home, I watched and waited for his car to drive into the school car park. I believed it was only a matter of time before he abducted me. I positioned myself near the windows and made sure I planned my exit route.

I would play out different scenarios in my head over and over again; what would I do if I saw his car?

Who would I tell?

What would I say?

What if the teacher didn't believe me?

Would I leave the class before he found me?

How? Would I explain to the teacher first or would I just run and hide?

What if he hurt the teacher?

What if he hurt the other children?

What if he had his shotgun?

Who would believe me?

How would I contact my mother? How would I find a telephone?

Would he be aggressive or would he be charming and persuasive? What would be better for me? I decided aggressive was best as if the teachers saw him for what he was, then they'd be more likely to protect me.

How would I escape?

If I didn't and he got me into his car, what would happen next?

This played out in my mind like a film until I was 16 years old, when leaving the constraints of formal education made me feel more in control of my own decisions and my own life. The fear stayed with me until adulthood. When I had my own children in school, I worried about them. I made sure that no one fitting his description was to be allowed to take my child out of school, but I was full of fear and felt impotent. When I spoke to the school staff I couldn't emphasise why this was so important because I still had no way of breaking my silence. I was frightened. Always.

At school it was exhausting to be in my head. I was tired. Sometimes I'd even fall asleep at my desk.

Some teachers were frustrated with me. I didn't listen. I couldn't keep up.

The older I got, the angrier I became. I was particularly angry with the male teachers. I also wanted their attention. Playing up resulted in negative attention which was satisfying as it was familiar and then justified my continued anger (in my head).

It never occurred to me to tell a teacher.

It never occurred to me to tell a friend. I didn't want them to know. It was my secret and I wouldn't have known how to tell. I thought that this abuser was the only one in the world like that and I was very ashamed of that.

I was seemingly a good actor because no one noticed this silent and awful private world inside my head and that continued to surprise me.

I remember feeling like most adults around me were actually quite stupid, which makes me sound arrogant, I suppose.

To: Pat
From: Sophie
I've sent you another story. I didn't write it before as I didn't think it was as important to put it down on paper. After our session yesterday though, this particular incident has played on my mind so there must be a reason for that.

Chapter 26

You're So Lucky

'You see now what has happened on account of your not listening to my counsel.'

– *The Golden Bird*, The Brothers Grimm

The Little Princess was standing in the playground, surrounded by a group of girls.

'Have you got a pony?' one girl asked the Little Princess, curiously.

The Little Princess hesitated. She looked at their faces. She could sense envy although she didn't know the word yet and was reluctant to answer.

'Have you?' said a second girl. 'A real pony? You're so lucky!'

And the Little Princess, seeing the wide smile on the girl's face, held her head up high.

'Yes,' she said with pride. 'I do. She's thirteen hands and four inches.'

'Aww!' chorused the girls. 'You're so lucky.'

'I wish I had a pony.'

'Can I come over to your house and ride her?'

'And me too?'

'And me?'

And the Little Princess felt that she was lucky and very special.

* * *

A few days later, the Little Princess stood in a field with the Big Princess and the Evil King. The Evil King was cross.

'You've missed some,' he said to the Little Princess. He looked her in the eye and she flinched, not wanting to become a Frozen Statue. 'Look!' he said quietly. 'What a stupid thing to do. It will be your fault if she dies. I'm disappointed in you. Look.' He was pointing at the yellow flowers left in the field. Ragwort. Ragwort, the Evil King had explained to the Princesses, would kill their pony if she ate it. He had made them listen as he described her slow death, the twisting of the gut, the blindness, the coma and pain, and now, with dismay, the Little Princess saw tell-tale yellow flowers and she knew she was a stupid and Useless girl to have missed them.

She felt the pressure of tears in her throat and tried to swallow them before the Evil King noticed.

'Go on!' he ordered. 'Go and pull them up. 'Hurry.'

And the Little Princess quickly walked away and let the tears fall but she kept her back to him and was careful not to make a sound.

She had been pulling plants from the ground all morning and her back and arms hurt. The roots clung with determination and the stalks ripped into the flesh of her palms and blistered her fingers as she pulled with all her strength.

The responsibility of her pony's life was a heavy burden to bear. She wanted to go home, and she wanted the Butterfly Queen. Holding the wilting ragwort in her arms, the Little Princess walked back to the Evil King, where he stood, arms crossed, and she placed the yellow plants in a pile with the rest.

The sun moved behind a cloud and the Little Princess shivered in the Shadow.

'Now we'll pick up the poo,' said the Evil King, putting on a large, stiff pair of gardening gloves and picking up a small shovel and a black bucket.

The Little Princess and the Big Princess stood and waited.

'What are you waiting for?' snapped the Evil King. 'Hurry up. There is a lot to do.'

'Where are our gloves and shovels?' asked the Big Princess.

'You can use your hands,' replied the Evil King.

And the Little Princess, as she knelt on the hard ground and picked up horse shit with her bare hands and put it in a bucket, understood that she wasn't special at all.

* * *

In Remove, the Little Princess sat at her desk and studied the crescent-shaped black shit under her fingernails.

'When can I come and see your pony?' whispered The Girl With The Wide Smile.

The Little Princess pretended she hadn't heard and The Girl With The Wide Smile turned away and smiled at someone else instead.

Exploring 'You're So Lucky'

To: Sophie
From: Pat
I have just read your next chapter, Sophie. So emotionally abusive to reduce you to grovelling on hands and knees, ensuring the possibility of friends was no longer a possibility for you . . . The pony could have given you hope, though if kids had come round, he may well have belittled you further in front of them. These memories are as important as the others . . . The build-up of guilt, feelings of uselessness and describing to you how the animal would die . . . more and more fear. He ruled with terror and fear.

To: Pat
From: Sophie
It made my world confusing. I was aware I was 'privileged' by my education and upbringing. Yet, I was treated like this. As a result, it made me feel separate from The World. I didn't feel like I really fitted in, with my private school peers or with children who lived in my village and went to the local state school. I'm not sure that many would identify though with this particular story, as a pony symbolises a lifestyle inaccessible to the majority. The irony of that doesn't escape me.

I've sent you a new one. Yesterday obviously released something.

Chapter 27

The Shadow of Rocks

'Then he flew down with her from the tree, and placed her on a daisy, and she wept at the thought that she was so ugly that even the cockchafers would have nothing to say to her.'
– Thumbelina, Hans Christian Anderson

The Little Princess's soul had been stolen and the Evil King had given her a Shadow in return. The Little Princess was tired of it. It had melded with parts of The Body and in those places, it burned and throbbed and the Little Princess couldn't shake it off, however hard she tried.

She tried laughing and playing in the garden of the cottage and sometimes bits of the Shadow would fall away as she played but the Evil King had placed a spell on the Shadow, making it belong to the Little Princess, and the bits would, without fail, make their way back to her.

This Shadow was heavy, as if made of giant rocks. The Little Princess was only small, and the weight made her little Body buckle with the strain. She worried she would not grow up to be tall and beautiful like the Butterfly Queen. *I shall surely grow twisted and crooked*, she thought. The Shadow of Rocks heard and thought this was a Good Idea and it shifted inside the Little Princess's Body until it found her bones. It wrapped itself around her spine and her small ribs, and its weight crushed and pulled and pushed and pressed until one day the Little Princess woke up and saw to her horror that her Body had indeed become twisted, and her bones jumbled up and bent. The Little Princess gasped in horror, but she couldn't take a deep breath. Her lungs were squashed, and her heart was inside a cage.

'Ha!' said the Shadow of Rocks.

The Evil King, far away in The World, heard the Shadow and was pleased.

'Ha!' said the Evil King.

The Little Princess was frightened. She needed to wait for her soul, so she fought against Growing Up.

The weight of her Shadow of Rocks that weighed her down, and the battle between her past and her future began to pull her in different directions and the Little Princess started to grow in different directions too, until her spine looked like an S instead of an I.

This made the Little Princess angry because she could see she had failed. She tried to stop her spine from curling, but she was too weak and stupid and it did it regardless.

The Little Princess knew that was getting what she deserved, for letting things go Wrong in the beginning.

Exploring 'The Shadow of Rocks'

Hi Pat. I feel like I'm losing a bit of the impetus.

Take a break now from it.

I wish that the fear and dread wouldn't come back so easily. One step forward. Two back.

That's quite usual and then one day something just flips, and you realise you just can't stagnate anymore.

My perpetrator is living and breathing. A psychopath.

Absolutely but even they can't live forever . . . and do you know what is wonderful . . . you have now acknowledged that that is what he is. 🙈

I've always known it. It's hard to speak though because I am part of him.

No, because you are the most wonderful mutation ever made . . . imagine how you might have turned out, but you didn't and it's unbelievable.

But I get scared and wonder if I'm conjuring up a demon by doing this. Don't think I have ever been called a mutation before 😊

Is He Really a Monster?

I've just sent you an email. It's what I was talking about last night in our session. It's a bit messy I'm afraid. It's a weird one, this one – I write and write and then I suddenly fall asleep. It's been one of the hardest ones so far even though it's relatively tame in comparison to some of the other chapters.

I will do a read-through later. It's probably hard because it's the young adult coming to a full understanding that there was no humanity to him at all. The memories fit together and confirm it. 'Normalisation' is an interesting process. Millions of people were killed by the Nazis in their homes, on the street and then in death camps, and it went on for years being 'normalised' by their population. I would like you to acknowledge that poor 14-year-old girl who only ever wanted to find love, and proof that her [perpetrator] was not really a monster.

Chapter 28

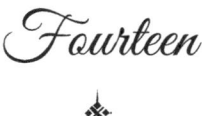

'Dear children, I have to go into the forest, be on your guard against the wolf; if he comes in, he will devour you all – skin, hair, and everything. The wretch often disguises himself, but you will know him at once by his rough voice and black feet.'

– *The Wolf and Seven Little Kids*, The Brothers Grimm

The Evil King had been away for four years. In the beginning, this was a relief for the Little Princess because the Shadow turned to Light and the family learned how to live. The Butterfly Queen and the Princesses learned how to laugh. They learned how to sing and how to dance and they slid across the tiled kitchen floor in their slippers and fell and laughed and sang and shrieked. The Evil King didn't hear because he was far, far away. The Little Princess was glad, and she was happy.

But Dark follows Light, and one day, the Little Princess awoke, and felt sad. Something very important was missing from her life. The Little Princess thought of other princesses and their Kings: Brothers. Uncles, fathers, grandfathers. Their Kings loved them. The Little Princess watched carefully as they gave their princesses affectionate hugs and played and laughed with them. The Little Princess worried she'd remembered everything wrong. She knew of the Big Black Door and the photographs and that SHE MUST NOT open it, but because it had been so long since she had seen him, she began to forget why, and thoughts of Snakes and Frozen Statues and Cold Ice Eyes began to fade from her mind. Sometimes, a photograph would escape, and the Little Princess would slide it back, face down, underneath the Big Black Door. She learned what made the photographs escape and consulted her list of Triggers, to remind herself how to stop it happening. She learned to check before walking up a flight of stairs in case there was someone behind her. She learned to avoid, and she learned how to Fear. She was careful and cautious as there were so many Triggers.

She learned to shut her eyes. Avoid. Not think. Avoid and exist, day after day, pretending that she was like the other princesses.

But she was Different. She could look in her mirror and it would helpfully reflect her twisted and bent Body, reminding her of quite how Different she was.

She said to the Butterfly Queen, 'I want to see You Know Who. I need him back. I want him,' and the Butterfly Queen was worried. She had been busy fluttering, but she wasn't stupid. She knew of the danger, and she was frightened for her Little Princess.

'Don't,' she said.' He's not safe.'

But she didn't tell the Little Princess why and the Little Princess was angry with the Butterfly Queen for being so vague. *If you don't talk about Snakes and Frozen Statues and Shadows, and I don't talk about Snakes and Frozen Statues and Shadows, then maybe they weren't real at all*, she thought.

'I can if I want, I can do what I like. You can't stop me,' said the Little Princess and of course the Butterfly Queen agreed. Because she couldn't stop her.

So, one terrible day, the Little Princess and the Evil King, met up once more.

The Little Princess got up, on this fateful day and she tried to make herself look pretty for the Evil King.

The Old Witch was back. *Grumble, grumble* went the Old Witch. *It's not safe. It's not safe. Stay here. Don't go. Stupid girl.*

'Shut up!' said the Little Princess, choosing baggier clothing to cover her twisted and bent Body. *You need to be pretty and perfect. Perfectly pretty and then he will love you*, she thought, and she checked herself from all angles, until she was satisfied that her Body was as hidden as it could be.

And the Butterfly Queen and the Little Princess drove out of The Kingdom and down the long country lane with the Little Princess's heart thumping in her chest.

Go back! Go back! grumbled the Old Witch, and the Little Princess turned up the radio to drown out the curses and shouts.

They parked in a busy car park in The World and the Butterfly Queen turned off the engine. They sat in silence for a moment or two, with the Little Princess's heart drumming so loudly that she was surprised The World couldn't hear it.

The Butterfly Queen asked the Little Princess if she'd reconsider and come home again but the Little Princess was stubborn, angry, and defiant.

'I want to do this,' she said. 'I want to see him.' And this was true. She was beginning to feel so much Fear, but she was also a little curious and she had hope. *Maybe,* she thought, *just maybe I have got it wrong.*

The Butterfly Queen looked as if she was going to cry.

'Please promise me,' she said. 'Don't get in the car with him.'

And the Little Princess felt two opposing feelings collide in her head. She felt a sense of pride. The Evil King wanted her and loved her so much that he wanted her to go and live with him, and she felt Fear. Overwhelming, stomach-lurching, skin-crawling Fear and it began to rise off her skin – little invisible whorls of delicious nectar that drifted through the open window.

'I promise,' she said to the Butterfly Queen. 'Do you think he will buy me a donut and a Coke?' she asked, and the Butterfly Queen didn't reply. She just looked sad.

Meanwhile, the Evil King, who was nearby, was feeling Powerful. His nostrils twitched as the smelled delicious nectar and he drank it in, greedily and lustily and was impatient with excitement. He hadn't been surprised when the Little Princess came to him. His expertise in Mind Capture was a force to be reckoned with.

He walked towards the sounds of The Little Princess's drumming, banging heart, to meet her once more.

They were to meet in the coffee shop and arrived at the same time. The Evil King was momentarily wrong-footed as the person standing in front of him was not quite as he'd remembered. She wasn't such a Little Princess.

The Little Princess was momentarily wrong-footed as there in front of her was the Evil King. But she couldn't see his Mask and they were in The World, so she felt confused. She could see his Ugly face. There was a gap where his front tooth had been, he was a Monster and he didn't even hide it. Beside the Evil King, stood a woman. She was small, with bright blonde hair and the Little Princess realised she was the new Queen. She implored silently to this Queen, *You'll keep me safe, won't you?* But when she glanced at her eyes, she realised in horror and disbelief that The Queen had Cold Ice Eyes.

Run away, shouted the Old Witch.

She dared to look at the Evil King, but his eyes weren't looking at hers. They were studying her Body and staring at the Little Princess's chest, where she was beginning to change and grow. He stared at her long legs. She could hear his breathing getting louder, and the whistle as it escaped through his nose. The Little Princess wrapped her arms around herself.

'Aren't you going to give me a hug?' he asked and he pulled her towards him and held her too close. It hurt her new breasts. The Little Princess felt like a rag doll and the Evil King gave her a kiss on the mouth and she tasted the saltiness of his Ugly, monstrous, slimy tongue as he pushed it inside her, just once, quickly. In, out, and the Little Princess gasped with the shock of it and wondered with her flaming face, how the people were still walking by and how they hadn't noticed.

Run! shrieked the Old Witch from inside the Little Princess's heart and mind, but the Little Princess didn't know how to run. Her legs were turning to Ice.

'Come on,' said the Evil King, 'let's go inside.'

So they walked inside and waited in the queue and the Little Princess's legs were shaking and she didn't know what to do but she knew she was in great danger.

She was shouting at herself, inside her head,

What have you done? You're so stupid! You never forgot at all! And she remembered it all. Cold Ice Eyes and Snakes and hurt and bites and she wanted to collapse right there in the middle of all these people drinking their coffee and smiling and chatting, and to fall asleep for a million years.

She couldn't of course. She stood, trapped. The Evil King had a firm grip of her hand and the Evil Queen stood close behind.

'Please can I have a Coke and a donut?' the Little Princess

asked but the Evil King didn't seem to hear. He ordered two coffees and two cakes, and a glass of water for her.

The Little Princess knew that the cakes weren't for her. She wanted to apologise for asking yet she couldn't speak. She felt ashamed as she knew she'd made the Evil King cross and she lowered her head.

They sat at the table. The Little Princess sat on one side and the Evil King and Evil Queen sat opposite.

The Little Princess sipped her water and waited for this awful day to end.

But, as it always did, things got worse and worse.

The Evil King took hold of the Little Princess's hands, and he held them gently and brought them to his face.

'I've missed you so much,' he said, and a tear appeared in his eye.

The Little Princess was bigger now and she knew it was a Trick. She waited.

He held her face and cupped her chin. 'Look at me,' he said gently, so the Little Princess had to look, and his Cold Ice Eyes locked into hers, whilst his hand gripped her face and she couldn't escape.

She could feel his fingers, as the Evil King started to caress her mouth. He rubbed them gently over her lips and The Little Trapped Princess remembered the Snakes. Then, she began to feel the Snakes. She could feel them prodding and crawling and pushing all over her Body, but of course, there was nothing there at all.

Help me, she said to The People, eating and drinking and chatting and laughing but only in her head so no one heard.

The Evil King heard her thought and it encouraged him to carry on with his assault because he enjoyed it even more when he could see her Fear.

The Little Princess saw a man, sitting nearby, who did seem to notice. He looked curiously at this trio and the Little Princess was ashamed.

Then, abruptly, it ended. The Evil King rose to his feet and the Evil Queen followed.

'It was your birthday, wasn't it? I have a present for you. It's in the car'.

The Little Princess began to panic.

Grumble, grumble went the Old Witch, and louder and louder went the thumping of her heart and she knew.

'I have to stay here,' said the Little Princess and her voice shook with Fear. 'the Butterfly Queen is meeting me here.'

'Well, we will have to be quick, won't we?' said the Evil King and with an arm across her shoulder, pushed her forward and out of the coffee shop, into the crowd and the car park and towards his car. The Little Princess stopped and watched as the Evil Queen got into the back seat and buckled up her seat belt.

Don't get in the car, whispered the Butterfly Queen and the birds and the Old Witch.

'Get in the car,' said the Evil King, as he got behind the wheel and secured his seatbelt.

The Little Princess watched the people in The World as they walked past, with bags of shopping and fruit from the markets. She wanted to scream, and shout HELP ME! but she couldn't move. She was a Frozen Statue.

The Evil King leaned across and flung open the car door.

The Little Princess saw he was angry.

'Get in the car,' screeched the Evil Queen, and the Little Princess hated her.

'Get in the car!' said the Evil King and the Little Princess remembered Hard, Wood Hands.

Stay out! Stay out! whispered the Old Witch, from inside the Little Princess's heart.

'Now,' he said, very quietly, and she could see that there was no choice. She sat down in the front seat. But she kept her legs out.

'Sit properly!
'Shut the door!
'Get in the car!
'Get in the car!
'Shut your door!'

And still the Little Princess didn't move. The Old Witch inside her heart was screaming and shouting and crying,

Stay out!
Don't move!
Stay out!
Stay out!
Help me!

Help me!
Where are you?

She was a Frozen Statue half in her old life and half in a new one, one that she knew led to pain and attack and she was so frightened she thought she would die from it.

But then, a curious thing happened. The thoughts subsided and quietened, and the Little Princess felt calm.

Her Body wasn't part of her anymore. Her legs belonged to The World and the rest belonged to the Evil King. She could feel the Evil King lean his heavy body across hers and she could feel him grabbing at her legs and pulling her seatbelt across her chest, but she was elsewhere. She was in the crowds of people with their fruit and their shopping. She was with the other families in the car park as they lifted small children out of car seats and placed them in pushchairs. She was at the ticket machine, watching as the coins clunked – one, two – and then she saw the Butterfly Queen and so did the Evil King and before she knew it, she was back with the the Butterfly Queen, driving up the country roads, back to the Kingdom and she had no idea how she had got there. She noticed that she was holding an envelope. With trembling hands, she opened the card.

To the Little Princess,
love from the Evil King.

She had survived.

Exploring 'Fourteen'

To: Sophie
From: Pat
So, I have read your email and it is very different. In this chapter, you are now able to comprehend what is happening but are still locked in fear. I like the end where you say, She had survived. And that's exactly what you have done. No more harming, Sophie, you have a story here that tells it all. This 'fairy story' will be so helpful and such a useful model for young people to use to express what has happened to them. Get out there and make a difference.
When we help others, we help ourselves. Then we recover and become so strong, nothing will break us. And then who knows what might happen to the monster. Imagine if you made it to TV and the press... you don't need to name him, but as you campaign for others and demand law changes, he will know that you haven't forgotten, and he will feel fear that one day they will come for him.

To: Pat
From: Sophie
I felt that I had survived something so huge and that I'd been moments from something, but it was never clear what. It was an attempted abduction which is going to be frightening for anyone. But life carried on. My mother was upset I had got in the car, that was it. I think I was really traumatised by that Saturday morning and never recovered from the fear.
What happened with [the perpetrator] that day felt the same as a brush with death I experienced later in life. Worse, because it was so prolonged.

To: Sophie
From: Pat
So, you were really meant to survive and now you must no longer dice with death.

To: Pat
From: Sophie
I need to still work on that fear. It's very strong today after writing that.

To: Sophie
From: Pat
Write down the fear, give it a voice and send it to me if you want. As you share it, it lessens . . . my fears are . . .

To: Pat
From: Sophie
I'm not sure how to. It's very physical.
I don't remember the accident I had with fear. I can remember the fear I felt at the time, but it doesn't make me fearful again. Or times of trauma from suicide attempts and being put in hospital. But I don't feel the fear now in the same way. But this, him . . . it's like my brain hasn't gone through the right processes or it's never been processed at all.

To: Sophie
From: Pat
Just take it gently. At the moment you are taking small steps. I hope you are not insulted by my use of the word mutation by the way. It's the only word I could find for something so transformative!

To: Pat
From: Sophie
No, not insulted in the slightest.
Made me laugh!

When I read stories about women, repeatedly beaten, abused and terrorised by their partners, who don't leave, or return to them again and again, I can understand why. The abuse ended when this man stepped out of my life when I was ten years old. Life was better. There was a sense of relief; the world seemed brighter. I felt like I could breathe again, at first.

When he wasn't there anymore, I felt this sadness inside me, because for the first time I began to dwell on what I'd lost. I looked carefully at my friends' relationships with the men in their own families, and I began to miss it, which was crazy because I hadn't ever had it. Our relationship was only ever about abuse. There was no kindness or love, just fear and shame.

I convinced myself that if I could see him again, it would be different this time and not as I'd remembered. I was determined that I was wrong, that I'd got it, and him, wrong. I refused to believe that it could happen again. That was then and this was now. I wasn't a child anymore (I thought) – I was older, wiser, nearly a woman. Someone he would be proud of. He would look at me and question how he could have walked away. He would love me when he met me again. I imagined the relationship we might have. Trips to the cinema. Maybe a holiday by the sea, where we would walk together, like normal people, and do what normal people do.

This thinking, this fantasy became my comfort blanket. I convinced myself that it would be true because I craved a normal relationship, and I made the fateful error of picking up the phone and calling him. Despite the fear of my mother who told me to forget it. Forget him. There was one big problem though; my mother didn't know about the abuse. It was hidden. Covert. It had mostly taken place in my house, more or less under her nose. Whilst she knew he was someone to be wary of, feared even, she didn't know exactly what he was capable of. No one did. Apart from him, and me. I think I shouted the words that teenagers often shout, something along the lines of, 'You can't tell me what to do!' and before long arrangements had been made and I was on my way to meet him.

What happened was so traumatic, it became part of my nightmares to be re-lived in thoughts, flashbacks and dreams for many years. It culminated in this attempted abduction that felt like one of the most dangerous situations I'd ever been in, yet must have been perceived by others as one of the most normal sights: an older caring relative, taking a young girl out for tea, on a Saturday afternoon.

He was the monster I'd forgotten. There was the same emptiness behind the eyes. The eyes. How could I have forgotten them? They filled me with fear. They always had. There was nothing there. A blank darkness. Years later J.K. Rowling's description of the Dementors in *Harry Potter and the Prisoner of Azkaban* – creatures that feed on a person long enough to reduce them to something like itself: soul-less and evil – would bring him to mind.

These eyes were looking at me once more. How could I have been so stupid and what would it take to get out of this alive? I remember the shock of his tongue that pushed quickly inside my mouth as he leaned in to give me a kiss. We were in a crowd of people, but no one noticed this brief assault. This was a deliberate reminder. It was a *'do you remember me?'*

As I described in the fairy tale, by the time I was in the coffee shop I was screaming out for help because I knew where this could lead, but no one heard the silent cries inside my head. Except one. The man, who sat on his own, reading his paper. I looked at him and he looked up at me. Then he looked away, and looked back again, and I could see the look of puzzlement on his face. He'd noticed that something was wrong with this picture. He kept glancing at us, and I stared into his eyes, desperate for him to do something, anything, to help me, but he ignored my silent plea and in the end, looked away.

I often thought of him, the man, with his coffee and his paper, and I wondered if he thought of me too. I wonder if he felt any guilt for turning away? He should have because **he knew**. He could see that there was something really wrong. He looked into my eyes and saw my terror and **he looked the other way**. I think about what I would do if I was in his shoes. Would I listen to my instinct and step up? Step in and confront? Would I ask the question, *'Are you OK?'* or *'Do you need help?'*

Or would I do the easiest thing of all – *normalise* and *rationalise* what I was watching because the alternative was a little bit too much trouble. Because it made me uncomfortable, awkward, and embarrassed? Because, what if I was wrong and I was shouted at, or worse? What if I made a fool of myself? Would my courage fail me? After all, it was nothing to do with me: it was not my business.

I'd like to think I'd do better.

Chapter 29

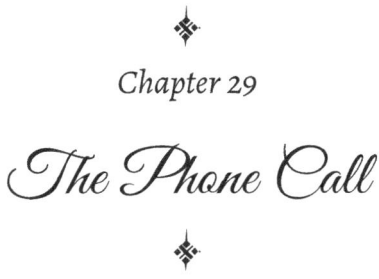

This is why whoever is not afraid of the devil can tear out his hair and win the entire world.

– Jacob Grimm

The Little Princess had her eyes closed as she held the phone against her ear.

She had told the Evil King she no longer wanted to see him, and she listened as he raged and ranted. Now the Little Princess understood that whilst she thought she'd seen the Evil King without his Mask, he'd been wearing another one underneath. Finally, this one was beginning to crack and fall away.

She saw him now.

She had never heard the Evil King speak with such anger. As she listened to his violent tirade, she imagined him, one hundred feet tall. A seething mass of wrath and fury. She pictured his heart. Small, shrivelled, and black. He was a Monster. Monstrous. She saw a demon, a devil, with a forked tail and horns on the top of his head.

'You are a whore, like your mother!' he shouted, and the Little Princess wondered how this would end.

She studied her bedroom. She looked at her teddy bear on her bed and tried to reach it, but she didn't know how to move her legs to get up from the chair.

'Cunt,' she heard the Evil King say.

Cunt, she mouthed silently, and wondered what the word meant. She twisted her hair around a finger.

C.U.N.T. She mouthed again, phonetically. It was a harsh word. It must mean something terrible. She was one.

The Phone Call

'What did you say?' yelled the Evil King
'What did she say?!' the Little Princess heard the Evil Queen screech in the background.
'Nothing,' said the Little Princess. 'Sorry.'
She wondered how her book could be waiting on her pillow and how her clothes could be neatly put out for tomorrow, when her world was turning upside down.

She could hear the Butterfly Queen, but she was far away, fluttering and flitting in another room in the house. She could hear the *thump, thump* of her sister's music, coming through the wall but the Little Princess was alone as she continued to listen.

She listened as the Evil King's vicious words surged along the phone line. They flowed into her ear and the sharp, guttural sounds pierced her heart. They shot along artery and vein and came to rest in the depths of the Little Princess's Body, infecting every part of her with their savageness and depravity. They settled in her memory, never to be forgotten.

The holes in her heart started to weep. The Little Princess's love for the Evil King began to leave her heart. Out it flowed, until there was nothing left, not even a drop, and the Little Princess felt a little lighter.

She listened as he threatened, intimidated, and coerced.

She listened and still it went on. The Little Princess felt she was caught in a trap, and that this would never end, but then it occurred to her she could, quite simply, hang up the phone.

Taking a deep breath, the Little Princess removed the phone from her hot ear. She watched her own hand tremble as it slowly placed it down.

Click.

And the Little Princess sat, still as a statue, his words throbbing inside her head, until day turned into night.

The Butterfly Queen came into her bedroom and found the Little Princess sitting in the dark.

'Are you OK?' asked the Butterfly Queen anxiously. 'How was the telephone call?'

The Little Princess looked at her mother and she knew that she would never know how to begin.

'What is a slut?' she asked.

* * *

By the end of her fourteenth year, the Little Princess's mind was finally full. Boxes and boxes of photographs stacked neatly in her mind.
    They became known as triggers.
Hands and
Gold rings and
Broad backs and
Fingers.
Fluffy chicks and
Wire fences and
Shiny shoes and
Fine clothes.
Snakes and
Suits.
The noise of cars and
Windows and
Darkness and
Light and
Headaches and
Kings and
Shadows and
Ice and
Eyes without lights and
Baths and warm water and
Whisky.
Cigarettes and
Rolled up sleeves and
Laughter and
Footsteps behind and
Staircases
And gloves.
Woods
And fields
And trees.
Black hair and
Jangling keys
And chewing
And breathing
And shouting
And

And
And
And, and.

Exploring 'The Phone Call'
How Strong My Voice Is When I Write

To: Sophie
From: Pat
I have read and sent back my comments. The phone call is the most brutal of all the chapters . . . it is both psychologically and sexually the most abusive thing I have ever read. I want to take that young girl and put her to rest in a crystal cave of love and light surrounded by animals and warm blankets.
Sophie, we so need that sanctuary of recovery for women with amazing therapists, holistic therapies and a small farm.

To: Pat
From: Sophie
We do. All we need is my book to sell as well as Harry Potter and then I'll set it up! Somehow, I don't think it will be quite as popular!

Did you feel that more strongly as a result of my writing? I ask because your response is a strong response, yet I think I've told you about that phone call before. I'm curious because if you're left with those feelings after reading my chapter, it shows the power of the written word, doesn't it?

It also shows how much stronger my voice is when I write, than when I speak.

If you remember me telling you about that call, how does that verbal account compare with the written one?

What is your opinion about the new chapters and if they would fit in the book?

To: Sophie
From: Pat
I will think about this over the weekend when there is more time. Yes, I remember the phone call but when someone talks about it, often they have learned to detach – they talk in a flat voice as if they are talking about a daily activity like shopping, for example. When written, it allows the reader their own interpretation and to absorb . . . more slowly . . . more powerfully. For example, they may read the piece over again, thinking, am I really reading this?!

I think that chapter is powerful because the child is now a young woman, and his disgusting venom is pouring out, attacking her femininity to the core.

To: Pat
From: Sophie
That's interesting. I think these stories should be documented, like the holocaust. It's not enough for them to be said privately in a therapist's room.

To: Sophie
From: Pat
Yes, the written word is lasting.

I began to wonder how others would react to my story. How powerful was the written word? If other survivors could relate to my fairy tale, would it encourage them to join me and to use their words to influence some sort of change? If the collective weight of these words reached The World, might it encourage people to stop putting the emphasis on there being something inherently wrong with adult survivors – struggling to live in a society that turns away from our pain, and instead begin to recognise our trauma and actively support us? I wanted to experiment and to gauge reactions, so began to carefully consider how I might share what I'd written, and with whom.

Working with Anger and Grief

At the same time, I experienced the most unexpected of all responses to the last two chapters.

There were many emotions released during therapy, anger being the strongest. This emotion I had turned on myself and I was learning to, with Pat's help, to reshape and redirect it at the Evil King, at what he'd done to me. Writing gave me permission to express this anger, but it was challenging because anger has always made me feel unsafe. I'm still frightened by it. It makes my heart gallop and adrenaline surge, and this feels too similar to panic. My instinct is to suppress or escape it with self-destructive behaviours – in the past, my go to response. Today I don't do that but there are times when I still really want to. Grief floored me at this point of my therapeutic journey. I shared my feelings with Pat in an email, after a therapy session, along with a letter I'd written to the Evil King as part of a writing task in one of my weekly writing groups.

To: Pat
From: Sophie
Subject: Feeling disconcerted
Hi Pat,
I have had the most disconcerting urge to contact [the perpetrator]. I haven't felt this for many years. The last time was when I was fourteen and I never ever expected to feel that again. It really unsettled me. I can see how women are pulled back to abusive relationships but in my case when I have been free of him physically at least, for so long, why do you think that could happen?

To: Sophie
From: Pat
OK, thank you for sending me this. What I would like you to do is spend some time to ask yourself 'why do I want to do this?' Make sure you listen carefully to the answer. The answer may well flow from your heart and the words may be very straight forward. It will possibly be the 'emotional you' speaking and that emotion can take any form.

**To: Pat
From: Sophie**
Why?
A few things come to mind.
When you're a child, your family home is an island. You look to the other islanders for guidance. You're young and you're impressionable. You copy what you see, and you do as you're told, because you are a child. You watch and absorb, and you adopt the traits, habits and behaviours of your parents and your siblings and anyone else who lives on that island with you.
Their accent becomes your accent. Your voice, their voice. Your mannerisms mimic theirs.
If they're open and generous and humble and kind, then that's what you become.
If they're mocking and intolerant, small minded and prejudiced, then you are too. If they put milk in the cup before the water, then you learn to put the milk in first. If they hold their knife like a pencil, it will never occur to you to hold yours in a different way.
You're a child and that is your job – to watch, learn, absorb, and adopt. You are not totally reliant though, you have your own instincts and morals and, if you're lucky, the islanders nurture these and encourage free thinking and growth. If you're unlucky, they stamp them out, insisting their way is the only way.
You may visit other places, other islands, but these visits are usually brief and before you know it, you're back on your island again.
Usually, as you grow, these visits become more frequent and, when you can, you save up the money to buy your own boat because you're a bit fed up with the islanders, day after day, and you outgrow them in the end. You crave more and you sail to the mainland where you meet many different people, ex-islanders with many different beliefs, behaviours, talents, opinions, accents and you begin to pick and choose. You take what you admire and they hold a mirror up to you, reflecting the bad and ignorant traits that you quickly discard in shame, as you learn the alternative and you grow, and one day you look back and realise the mainland is another country to the one you grew up in and that you can hardly understand the language anymore when you go back to visit.
[The mainland} was life and for my first ten years [the perpetrator] was the most important person of all because he

held it all in his hands as he was the most powerful. Then one day, [the perpetrator] left and my life shattered. He was the most important person but also the most cruel and unkind person, so we had to celebrate his leaving to make him the most unimportant person, reduced to nothing more than something unpleasant found on the bottom of a shoe.

But there was no room for loss. There was no room for grief because he was insignificant, revolting, dangerous, cruel, a bully, a coward, unkind, unloving, uncaring, destructive, a shit, a bastard, and how can you grieve for a man like that? So, the sense of loss for someone who had hurt me so appallingly was very profound because he was my most important person, but I wasn't able to express it, ever.

I have never grieved for that loss and for [the perpetrator].

To: Pat
From: Sophie
I wrote the letter to him as part of a writing homework task, and I said a lot of things in that but I suppose I never said goodbye. I don't know how I'm supposed to grieve for him, I certainly don't know how to grieve for myself.

I think my mask of bricks was a suit of bricks too. My mask has been chipped away, brick by tiny brick but the bricks on my body remain, particularly around my heart. It's bricked up and trapped and I think my soul is in there too. I want to remove these bricks and I need my emotions back, but I'm terrified of emotion because of where it leads me. I feel emotion when I drink and it swallows me up, leaving me in a very dark place. I can't go back there anymore.

The other part is harder to express.

I think it's to do with anger but I'm unsure. My feelings still don't feel like my own and I struggle to identify what I feel at all.

If I am able to begin to care for myself rather than harming myself, I am left with anger and frustration. It's not there all the time but it ebbs and flows, triggered by events that take me back.

I suppose I struggle then to see myself as worthy because I think I'm weak when I should be strong. By contacting him, I'm putting myself into a situation where I'll be hurt and abused again which I believe he would do, but maybe that is what I deserve because I'm not worthy enough to heal.

It's a really twisted view of this and I don't feel this all the time

– in fact, I'm feeling positive about where I am in the therapy, but it's definitely there in me.

To: Sophie
From: Pat
Yes, all varieties of emotions are coming into play here and we can talk them through. Meanwhile writing about it more fully might help. And you are right, you never got to say goodbye and this might be something you need to voice. In your 'letter 'to him (explored in therapy session) you asked him lots of questions but what do you want to tell him?

Chapter 30

Repercussions: Sleeping Sickness

'Oh, how silly of me! I've pricked my finger!' And the very next second she had fallen asleep, there, all amongst the dust, in her wonderful party dress, and her bright little crown!

– Sleeping Beauty; The Treasury of Fairy Tales,
Hilda Boswell

One morning, when the Little Princess opened her eyes, she knew something was wrong with her Body. She sat up in bed and she tried to stand up, but she couldn't. Her legs were filled with rocks and stones. She tried to wipe the sleep from her eyes, and she saw that her hands were filled with rocks and stones too and the effort was so great that she lay back down in her bed and went back to sleep.

The hours passed and the Butterfly Queen noticed that the Little Princess hadn't appeared for breakfast, so she fluttered upstairs to the Little Princess's bedroom and peered at her sleeping face.

'Wake up!' she said. 'It's late. Come downstairs.'

The Little Princess, again sat up in bed and again tried to stand, but her Body was too tired and weary.

'I will call The Doctor,' said the Butterfly Queen, and the Little Princess said *no*, but only in her heart as she was too tired to make the words come out. She fell asleep again, tossing and turning with the fever that had taken control and had bad dreams about Snakes and Shadows. She woke to find strange male Hands touching her Body and the Little Princess froze in an instant.

The Doctor felt her head and her neck and prodded and probed and the Little Princess felt herself shrinking. His Hands moved along her Body. He felt her breasts and under her arms and between her legs and the Little Princess disappeared completely. She didn't think she was there at all, but then she heard their voices. She was wrong.

'What a Good Girl,' said The Doctor.

'What a Good Girl,' said the Butterfly Queen.

But the Little Princess wasn't Good. She had Bad thoughts. She was full of Fear and anger and rage and she hated The Doctor who had come into her bedroom and sat on her bed and touched her Body without even asking. If she'd had a knife, she would have chopped off each finger and stabbed him through his heart. Instead, she waited until she was alone and curled up into a tight ball and fell asleep.

She slept and she slept, and she slept.

The days turned into weeks.

'We're not sure what's wrong,' said The Doctor, coming back again, stealing her blood and taking it away with him in little glass vials.

The Little Princess thought she was dying. She didn't really mind because she was too tired, and death would mean she could sleep forever so she waited for it to arrive.

When the Darkness Descends

To: Sophie
From: Pat
Of course, the doctor had no idea what was really going on for you. In those days doctors never asked children or young people for their permission to examine them or even to explain what they might be doing and why. I am assuming your mother stayed throughout the examination. What was wrong with you?

To: Pat
From: Sophie
I had glandular fever. Yes, she did stay.

On a separate occasion I went to see a consultant and I tried to resist the examination. I remember him saying, "Don't be coy," and then getting cross and saying to my mother, "Can't you tell her to behave herself?" I was 14/15.

She was very upset and apologised to me afterwards. She explained that she was frightened because she didn't know what was wrong with me. She acknowledged he shouldn't have spoken to me like that.

I was so ill that I couldn't go back to school and missed almost my entire fourth year.

It took me a long time to recover. I was then diagnosed with ME/CFS (myalgic encephalomyelitis or chronic fatigue syndrome) and had recurring tonsillitis. I was about 20 before I felt like myself again but by then my scoliosis had deteriorated so badly that I had something else to worry about.

My body has always felt like it doesn't really belong to me. I am very detached from it as it has always let me down. Apart from pregnancy. Then I loved it but unfortunately, I couldn't stay pregnant forever!

Adulthood

To: Pat
From: Sophie
Hi Pat,
I think in my story there is a big gap between the teenage Little Princess and the pregnant/ married princess and that this chapter is very important for my continued work in therapy. I wonder if there are many other survivors like me, who don't reach and fulfil their dreams and potential because of the abuse that they suffer and the cruel words that they hear and believe about themselves, that turn into vicious self-doubt. I'd love your feedback, if possible, as a reader and as a therapist.

Later on that night Pat responded . . .

To: Sophie
From: Pat
Hi Sophie,
Yes, it is usual for people to believe that because they have been told they will never do anything in life or achieve anything. Often, they then go on and fulfil the prophecy. The negative words become a mantra and build into a belief system, and the work we do in therapy tears away these negative words and false beliefs. This is the hard work we are doing together. I will answer this more fully later.

To: Pat
From: Sophie
Thank you. I hope you've had a good day.

Chapter 31

The Person In Charge

'I am not safe; let me go away with people who will give me the sympathy I need so much.'
'I fear such people are very seldom to be found in the world.'

– *The Maiden Without Hands*, The Brothers Grimm

When she was nineteen, the Little Princess left The Kingdom of His to study far away, at University. She felt that her life was finally beginning, and she was excited about who she would become.

She hoped the Shadow of Rocks would stay behind in The Kingdom of His, but to her disappointment found it remained firmly attached and the Little Princess had to hide behind a bigger and stronger Mask, because she was ashamed and didn't want others to see her Shame.

The Little Princess sat in cavernous lecture halls and tried to listen and to learn and to become Someone New but she was distracted by the heavy Masks and she felt tired. She tried to listen, but the lecturer's words were too fast, and the Little Princess didn't have the energy to keep up. She tried to concentrate but all she wanted to do was sleep.

One morning, the Little Princess awoke to find the Shadow of Rocks sitting on her chest. She tried pushing it off, but it curled itself tightly around her arms and wrists and she remembered a thousand writhing snakes. She considered fighting the Shadow but then she saw her Mask in the corner of the room and she heard the Old Witch grumble, *What's the point?* and the Little Princess was so exhausted at the thought of the day ahead, that she closed her eyes and went back to sleep instead.

The next day was the same and the Little Princess didn't get out of bed, and she didn't shower either.

On the third day, the Little Princess decided she must eat, but the Shadow of Rocks sat in her stomach like a stone and there was no room for food, so the Little Princess closed her eyes and went back to sleep.

The days went by, and the Little Princess slept. When she was asleep, she didn't see The World, the Big Black Door or the Shadow of Rocks. When she was asleep, she didn't feel the Fear and The Shame, but when she woke up, her heart danced and jumped and leaped with Fear at the thought of the day ahead and the Little Princess didn't feel strong enough to face it, so she didn't. She gave in and she gave up and instead, she slept and slept and slept.

By the end of the fourteenth day, the Little Princess saw that she had no choice, and if she was to study and learn and become Someone New, she must get some help. So, with a huge effort and a muster of courage she went to find The Person in Charge.

She knocked on the door and looked at The Old Lady standing in front of her with relief. *Old ladies are kind*, thought the Little Princess, and taking a deep breath, began to speak, doing her best to explain the Shadow of Rocks and why she'd been sleeping for fourteen days and fourteen nights and how she hadn't been able to keep up with the words, but her voice shook and it was hard to know what to say at all so her words tumbled out, upside down and inside out.

'Stop!' snapped The Old Lady and she berated and criticised and scorned and mocked the Little Princess who saw that she had got it wrong. This wasn't a little old lady at all, she was an Evil Witch, wearing an old lady Mask. the Princess was beginning to learn that mask-wearing was commonplace in The World.

'I'm sorry,' whispered the Little Princess, desperate to escape from The Evil Witch and her harsh words but The Evil Witch hadn't finished. She put a curse on the Little Princess.

'You will never achieve anything,' she spat. 'You will never be a success, you will be a drain on society, you will never be welcome at another university, you are a disgrace,' and she told the Little Princess to leave.

    And the shamed Little Princess believed The Evil Witch as she had heard these words before. Doing as she was told, as she always had, the Little Princess stepped out of the room and off the wheel of life she had been travelling on and she watched as the rest of The World carried onwards and upwards without her, taking her future with it.

Chapter 32

Repercussions: Grey

'Who in the world am I? Ah, that's the great puzzle.'

— Alice In Wonderland, Lewis Carrol

Many years passed by. The Little Princess married a Kind and Beautiful Prince but felt very lonely as she spent much time in her mind which was full of Secrets and photographs. She had built a door years before, painted it black and kept it locked and bolted, so she didn't have to look at the photographs, but she knew they were there. Sometimes, one would find its way out and it would slide under the gap of the Big Black Door, and she couldn't help but glance at it as she slid it back underneath. The knowledge of the room behind the Big Black Door and the glimpses of the photographs manifested as a deep sadness inside her. Gradually, the colours of The World began to fade away until the Little Princess could no longer see the bright blue of a summer sky or the yellow of a daffodil or the pretty pink blossom on the trees. Everything was now a varying hue of Grey, as if she were not only dragging the Shadow of Rocks behind her but living inside the Shadow itself. Colour, for the Little Princess, had disappeared entirely.

She didn't tell anyone that colour had disappeared in case they thought she'd lost her mind or asked her why, and she became a great actor.

'Look at that beautiful rainbow!' she'd exclaim loudly. 'What a vibrant red rose!'

And no one seemed to notice she was pretending.

One day, when the Little Princess got out of bed, she saw a transparent bubble had appeared in the night and she was inside it. She tried to step through the bubble, but it moved with her, remaining firmly one inch in front. *What will people think of me inside this bubble?* thought the Little Princess, but soon discovered that not one person noticed it was there. They carried on talking to the Little Princess and she carried on with her strange, Grey life, trapped inside this clear cage.

To: Sophie
From: Pat
You are well on the way to recovery. He was darkness and you are the light and that's what he could not cope with. He wanted to destroy your beauty and light. Do not doubt your light. It is there, strong, and beautiful and it will shine in spite of him.

It is no wonder you could not relate to anyone. Who could begin to comprehend what you had lived with all these years? It's akin to being a prisoner of war. You were a child without the adult mind to understand that he was the sickness. He should have been in Broadmoor.

Triggering Event

Autumn

Pat and I received devastating news that one young girl from the peer support groups had died by suicide. She was the third survivor of Child Sexual Abuse I knew to take their own life and Emma's death had a profound and serious effect on me. It made me reflect on how many of us don't survive. The definition of the word survivor is, *A person who makes it out alive from an event in which others have died.*

Emma's death was a triggering event, and my mood began to plummet. I began to dwell on suicide and why I was still alive when others weren't. I had the sense that suicide was an inevitable outcome.

> **I'd like to dedicate any work I do to Fran, who died as a result of abuse.**
>
> Yes, I agree that the world needs to know those who don't make it through. Numbers are very high.
>
> **If I make it through, then I'll make sure of it. That's not meant to sound dramatic. It's the reality. I hope to find continued strength every day, because I need to make a difference.**
>
> There comes a time when you know you can't quit because the mission becomes too important. It becomes easier to go on, than to leave without completion, if that makes sense.
> **Yes, that makes sense. I'm struggling tonight but I know tomorrow will be easier. It usually is. It's about holding on when you feel you can't. It's like being a small boat in a vast ocean with no anchor, sail, or motor. When the sun comes out again, you're OK.**
> **Good night. Sleep well xxx**
>
> You too. Take care xx

The next day . . .

> As I went down old and familiar paths yet again last night, I realised that it's just a slow suicide really and I had a sense that it must be the last time. My body and mind today feel totally wrecked and I'm so tired. I am finding it very very hard.

Sometimes we must go into the void before we can let it go. Many people call it 'the dark night of the soul'. Then we emerge from it and self-destruction has no place in our lives anymore.

> **I feel I've had too many times where that's happened. I don't understand why I'm still here and others are not . . . Or why I can't put a final stop to this.**

With therapy, where would you like to go next with it? What needs processing and sorting next? What would you like to study/do next?

> **I am focusing on my writing when I can. I want to set up The Flying Child as an organisation but am unsure of how to at the moment. I'm hoping that will become clearer to me.**
> **I want to carry on with the therapy in tandem with all of this because I need to stop slipping backwards and perhaps that's one thing that will stop me doing that.**
> **I just don't want to keep going backwards!**

So, what is backwards for you? Look at the root cause of going back . . . why would you want to go back . . . what do you need to be in the moment . . . what do you need to move forward . . . deeply analyse these.

> **OK. I'll do that. I know that I don't want to go back.**
> **CSA needs a movement behind it and men involved too, but where do I go with the workshops in schools? Or do you think my time would be wasted on these? Does it depend on who we are trying to educate?**
> **For example, if the message to schools is that the child stops being a victim of CSA once childhood ends or the abuse**

stops, then could that trivialise the abuse? The reality is dysfunctional, chaotic lives and often death. The focus of these workshops would be the silence. Why are people silent about this? How can we challenge this?
It feels like there is so much to do but I know we have to start with something.

Yes, it is about breaking the silence. This needs to happen in school and that is where your heart lies. Follow your gut instinct on all of this and it will tell you what your role is. Workshops are needed for adults working in education and, indeed, everyone working with children. Once people are aware that CSA happens in their own communities and sometimes on their own doorstep, this will bring change. Focus on your part . . . it is a bit like cleaning up the planet . . . one group tackles the plastics . . . another the transport . . . one tackles recycling . . . another conservation. We need a network of people too.

I'm not sure what my gut instinct is but I know it is to do SOMETHING!
And I know it's to do with fighting silence. I keep coming back to workshops, but I wouldn't want them to just be in schools. It would be about adapting them for different areas in society.

This is now focusing time . . . go to your inner truth for this. Trust what you needed as a child when you were young. You came with special gifts. You knew what was happening to you, but nobody listened . . . what would you have needed in place for them to listen . . . brainstorm it . . . write it out and refine it.

I feel like I need to tell my story. For people to recognise what they see is not necessarily truthful. To look beneath the surface and to listen to instinct. I feel my story can help do that . . .
But . . . is that the wrong thing to do? Is my story too much about me when the focus should be on collective abuse?
Or . . . do I start with me but bring others in as well? It's difficult. I don't feel the same sense of urgency from others to do what I want to do. People respond half-heartedly and

that's not good enough. I need another me. I can't do it on my own because my instinct is that it needs more than me and more power behind it.

Yes, it does. It depends whether you still fear to tell your story?

No, I don't fear telling my story. I think it's important to tell it.

OK so now ask yourself how and where?

Everywhere. Why not?

But still I continued to struggle. I found this period of time the most frustrating of all because I truly believed I had left this darkness behind, and my focus was now on setting up The Flying Child and publishing the book. It was devastating to feel I was back at square one, wrapped in the Shadow, and unable to believe in a better tomorrow. I slipped backwards to old coping mechanisms and at one point considered ending my life. It felt like I was dying anyway. Suicide felt an inevitable consequence of Child Sexual Abuse.

Hi Pat, sorry for the delay. I'm not doing as well as I should.

It's so good to hear from you. I always get very concerned with silence. All you can do is the best you can do.

My best doesn't keep me safe from harm. I didn't want to wake up on Tuesday morning but I did again, but I don't understand how, and I don't understand how I get to these terrible places so fast and I just want it all to stop. I could feel it coming and I messaged you, but I deleted it.

I saw you had deleted the message. Keep communicating at this time. It's really important.

I don't know what to say anymore.

Just keep going and when you can, throw your feelings into your book and get it finished. Start to think about marketing.

Keep focused because without focus we have no purpose. When we work on helping others, we ultimately help ourselves.

I can't do that when I'm being pulled back. The pull is so strong, and I feel like I'm dying. I wonder if I'm already part way there – not my physical body but my soul. I feel the pull in the opposite direction too, which is purpose and living but the dying bit has become so strong. I don't fear it anymore. I need guidance to stay here but my family will only see one type of guidance which isn't one I can or will accept now. I feel in my heart that it's the wrong choice to go now but I don't know how to stay. How do I find help?

You find help going within to the stillness. Let go of all of this . . . should I stay, or should I go? and just be . . . with no judgement about it . . . no expectations just simply be in the moment . . . neither in the past nor the future because then we never experience the now. Your past is done . . . you can't change it so work with what you have now.
This period will pass, and we just have to learn from it. The most difficult times of our lives give us the maximum growth. It's what we choose to do with that growth and learning. First, we help ourselves and then we move outwards. And so it goes on from there.

I know the consequence on others. That's the only answer my psychiatrist gives me and that's why I'm still here, but if I was a dog, I would be put to sleep. Because my behaviour will have far-reaching effects on my children is why I should go. I'm weak and selfish because I can't snap out of it this time and I don't want them to see me like this, but I don't know what to do to help myself. Not in this situation. I am trapped. I'm sorry. Thank you for your reply, but I know it's impossible for anyone to help me other than me. I'm really sorry to have asked you.

Don't be sorry. I have just helped you to reinforce what the answer is. You know, Sophie, deep down psychiatrists, me, medication, harming . . . none has the answer. The only answer is to find a depth of strength within you to survive through this.

It will give my children the ability to live more naturally in this unnatural world and to be free from this darkness that is inside me because it was passed on to me. I break the pattern and that is then the gift. I know medication is not the answer. Going back to the hospital is not an option either. You said keep communicating. If you didn't mean that, then please say. But I know from experience that I don't feel like that about suicide when I'm OK. When I was OK and I read my diary from before, when I felt like this, I couldn't understand how I felt like it would be OK for my children, and I believed I'd never feel these things again. So why do I now feel this again and how do I find the depth of strength? I want to be a good mother to my children. But this isn't good enough.

Being the best mother you can be is all you can do. Connect back with your inner child. She is frightened and alone and so becoming chaotic. She is screaming out and no one is listening. Ask her what she wants, but you probably instinctively know as a mother what that is already. Play with your child . . . have fun making pictures . . . not just about the book . . . but magical pictures just for the joy of it.

I don't understand. What child do you mean?

Yours inside YOU.
Left all alone back in the darkness.

That is what I wrote. I wrote it as the Little Princess to try and explain it, a few days ago.

Chapter 33

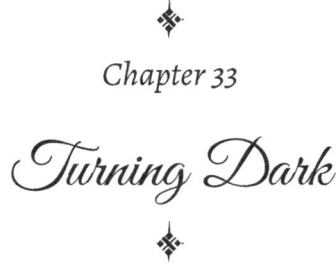

Turning Dark

"She had a little house of her own, a little garden too, this woman of whom I am going to tell you, but for all that she was not quite happy."
— Thumbelina, Hans Christian Anderson

The World was turning Dark. The Little Princess stood still, in the middle of a room in the middle of her house. It was the middle of the day, but when she looked out of the window, she could see that the sun had disappeared and the sky was Dark.

Then the Little Princess went to another window to look for the light, but she could only see the Darkness.

She opened the front door, and The Dark began to creep inside, so she slammed it shut quickly.

It was too late. The Dark had latched on to the tips of her toes. The Little Princess's feet were ice cold. She felt The Dark crawl up her feet and legs and body and down her arms and into the ends of her fingers. She felt it slide into her ears and her mouth and across her eyes. She felt The Dark anchor in her bones and settle deep inside her heart. The Little Princess became The Dark and The Dark became the Little Princess.

The Darkness made The Little Princess terribly cold, and her Dark soul began to shiver and shake.

She decided to ignore it. Perhaps lighting the fire would warm her cold body. Maybe she would find some light in the flames. But when she tried to lift her arms to strike the match, she couldn't. The Darkness that enveloped the Little Princess was viscous and it felt like moving through thick treacle.

There's no point, whispered The Dark in her ear. *The flames will die and the darkness will still be here.*

She turned on her television to look for the light but she saw Dark shapes and Evil people and conflict and hatred and abuse. She saw that the whole world had turned Dark and sick. She heard The Darkness in her heart whisper, *But you knew that already.*
She thought about making herself a cup of tea.
There's no point, said The Dark inside her stomach. *All that effort for the few minutes it will take to drink it.*
She tried to sleep.
There's no point, said The Dark behind her eyes, *because when you wake up in the morning, I will return.*
The Little Princess knew she could not live without light and she told The Kind and Beautiful Prince about The Dark. She hoped that if she spoke about it, The Darkness would be released, but it didn't work. Instead, she heard her words: how Ugly and Dark they were, and she saw how they frightened The Kind and Beautiful Prince, who was still able to see the light. He didn't know how to help her.

'Just keep going and never look back,' whispered the Little Princess to herself. 'Who needs light anyway?' And the Old Witch watched silently from afar.

Exploring 'Turning Dark'

Are you still feeling like this since we have talked? Have you managed to go out for a while yet and see beyond the dark outside the front door?

Yes. After a few false starts. I'm experiencing panic like I never have before, when even opening the door. If someone rings the bell, I feel the same. I'm not exercising enough so I'm restricting my food intake because I feel I'm not using enough calories but I'm also not feeling hungry anymore. At least I got dressed for the half an hour I was out.

There are times when we must push ourselves or we retreat back into a shell that's hard to get out of. You might enjoy yourself if you give yourself permission to do so. It's important to keep focused on life and do what we can with it.

I feel like an animal in the headlights of a car and that any extra pressure right now could push me to a dangerous place. I am not myself.

Then it might be time to talk with your psychiatrist to get something to take the edge off this fear.

I don't think suicide is easy. I think if it was, I would have gone. I have an inner turmoil and the pull to stay. My children.

So eventually you will reach the conclusion that it is not your time to go, because there are better things to do with thoughts than using them to find ways of quitting. Every ounce of energy is needed to raise a family and to do the job you have been sent to do. Xx

I hope so. I thought I had reached that conclusion but here I am. I am in so much pain.

You will eventually get there because soon your desire to 'get the job done' becomes greater than the wish to quit.

Please can we talk again some time?

Later that day . . .

To: Pat
From: Sophie
Dear Pat,
This is hard to put into words but please bear with me.
    I want to live. I want to live a normal, good, and productive life.
    I wanted to be a mother and I am. I think I have been a good enough mother, but not a perfect one. I want to live for the best part, but I have moments when I don't. This is one of those moments. I don't want to live but I still want those things and I'm still a mother. How can I want both?
    So, what I'm wondering now, is, what if suicide is part of my destiny, even if I don't really want it? What if that's just the way I have to die, even if I don't want to go?
    What if that's why I am always pulled back to suicidal thoughts, even when I feel my life is going OK?
    What if I need to stop fighting, like you said, but stop fighting to live, and fight to die?
    What if this was always part of my journey, and my children's journeys, for reasons that will become clear once I go?
    How would I ever know? Why am I always pulled back to this when all I really want is to live a good, normal, and productive life?

To: Sophie
From: Pat
We will talk about this tomorrow and of course we have a choice. Life only gets so much easier when we stop fighting it and go with the flow of it, enjoying every minute and not looking back and not looking forward. Suicidal thinking is suppressed anger, where destruction parades itself as being the only answer. Logically no one would really want to die by suicide unless they knew they were going to be killed and couldn't escape or had a terminal illness.

To: Pat
From: Sophie
It probably doesn't make sense, what I'm saying. It does in my head.

My children make me laugh. My son said today that sleeping wasn't sleeping, it was just 'one long blink'.
And then he farted in the bath and said he had made his own bath bomb.

Exactly – that's what you wanted in life – to be a mum in spite of what the monster did to you . . . and you don't yet know where this will all go.
I was once told that in the end, it is not the story that is important, it is what you do with it .
You have your story. What do you want to do with it now?
I know many people will benefit from what you can do. Your kids will have their mother to look up to. You are so talented in art and writing. You can potentially make a good life for yourself financially too.

Winter

To: Pat
From: Sophie
So tonight, I feel like an old car. One that struggles to fire, but then you pull the choke and press just the right amount on the accelerator and then it comes to life. Then it drives along quite happily, and you're looking forward to the rest of your day, and not backwards to where you'd be remaining static, if the car hadn't started. But then you hit a crossroad and it's no big deal, you've negotiated this many times a day for as long as you can remember, but the car stalls. Inexplicably. You had been driving OK and there's no reason for it to have stalled, but it has.

My psychiatrists would call this rapid cycling, hence the diagnosis of bipolar. Life can feel full of purpose and light and then an hour later you're back down in the dark, with their ugly face in your mind and the feel of their hands on your body and you can't shake it off.

To: Sophie
From: Pat
This is all quite normal when we have survived on the fumes of negative experiences for most of our lives. We get to the point where we 'miss' it because it is so much part of our whole being. So, when we leave it for a while, and we trundle along and life looks good, the unconscious reminds you, 'Hey, who are you to be living this great happy life? Do you remember how you were before, because do you know what? That is really who you are.'

And so, the internal monologue begins again, and the old patterns come back. The psychiatrists call it 'bipolar'. I don't quite see it that way. I compare it to tense, stiff muscles that you keep negotiating with, until the years of stress slowly peel away, and the muscles gradually realign themselves to a new way of being.

And then in the middle of summer, we suddenly get a day where we remember the cold and dark of winter and we may spend a day dreading its return and this is all OK. It's part of life. It's never all wonderful all the time but it's much better than the dark of the past where this awful monster lived for a very long time. And as we go on dealing with this monster and his behaviour and we help others with the same difficulties... The world grows lighter. You will notice this when you are out there, putting into action all the wonderful things that you have prepared.

* * *

I've just written a new chapter – a new one about birth. It's the only one that the process of writing has made me cry. It's frightening to feel such strong feelings. Please can I send it on?

Yes, send it on.

Chapter 34

'It's no use going back to yesterday because I was a different person then.'
— Alice In Wonderland, Lewis Carrol

More years passed, and the Little Princess got used to living in The Dark. She married her Prince, and on her twenty-second birthday, the Princess looked in astonishment as a second pink line appeared like magic, in the window of a white plastic stick.

She was pregnant and she waited impatiently for the days to pass and for the day that she could hold her daughter. The labour was violent and bloody. The Little Princess was frightened to release her precious child into a world of Shadows and Snakes, so the baby remained stuck, until with determined fingers, the midwives coaxed and pulled at the baby, but to no avail.

'We will have to transfer you to hospital,' they said.

'No,' said the Little Princess and with fierce effort and a muster of courage, she pushed her child out. She held the slippery little creature on her chest and watched with amazement as it turned into a little pink bawling baby, who promptly lifted her little head and looked around the room with large blue eyes.

'She's strong,' remarked The Midwife.

'You're like me,' the Princess, who was no longer Little, whispered to her daughter and her daughter opened her mouth to reply but clamped it over her mother's nipple instead and began to suck with furious determination.

The Princess wondered if maybe this had been The Purpose of her life all along.

Her Body worked for the first time. It may have been

twisted and bent and she may have been tired and weighed down by the Shadow of Rocks, but she could still make a baby. Her Body could keep it safe and let it grow. She could give birth and her breasts could make milk. the Princess had never felt so powerful and when the months had passed, she decided to do it again.

'Do you want to know the sex of the baby?' asked The Doctor and the Princess was surprised. She felt uneasy and she couldn't decide so the doctor wrote it on a piece of paper and sealed it in an envelope and the Princess and her Kind and Beautiful King took it home.

One day, the Kind and Beautiful King went out to buy some milk and curiosity got the better of the Princess. She knew it would be a girl, but she felt unsettled, and wanted to check just in case.

She opened the large brown envelope and removed a large sheet of white paper.

Male.

A little word. Four letters. Written at the top of the page and the Princess collapsed to her knees. She felt herself shrinking and the Big Black Door in her mind unlocked and swung open and there was nothing she could do about it. She remembered the Snakes. the Princess lay on the floor and curled up into a ball, but she felt the Snakes anyway.

She felt the bruises and the bites and the flicking tongues.

She felt the hard fist in the small of her back and the salty tongue taste in her mouth.

She shook with Fear as she remembered the Darkness and the Cage and the Turning Out The Lights day.

She had been so wrong. Her Body was stupid and Useless and had betrayed her by making A Male. The Evil King had tricked her again. He was back, a part of him, flesh and blood, this time, living and growing inside her own Body and the Princess wanted it out.

The poor Kind and Beautiful King came back with the milk and didn't know what to do.

He found the Princess, punching her stomach, screaming and crying with Fear and rage and didn't know how to help her. He heard her words and tried but couldn't understand as he'd never seen Snakes and Shadows. Neither could the poor

Midwife, who did her best to understand and held the Princess close, whispering reassuring words about little boy babies and telling her repeatedly that it would be alright. She said if the Princess's Body were made of glass, she would see a beautiful boy baby, gentle and loving and kind, like his father, not an Evil King at all, but the Princess didn't believe her. Her heart was full of hate and she hit her stomach every day. She was too cowardly to go to The Doctor and have the child ripped from her womb, so she waited in Fear for the day that the Monster would be born and then she would give it to someone else.

One night, the Princess woke up. Her Body was trembling all over. She shook and shook and wondered why. She didn't feel cold. The Monster was due, and she didn't even feel Fear anymore as she knew she'd soon be rid of it. She went back to sleep and soon after she awoke again, this time with a violent contraction that gripped her Body in a vice. She screamed out in pain and woke her Kind and Beautiful King.

'It's coming,' she said, and she'd barely spoken before, again, she writhed in tortuous agony as the contractions came fast, tearing her Body apart and hardly giving her time to breathe.

She retreated to a dark room and backed into a corner, tearing out a chunk of her own hair in her pain and distress and began to birth her baby, screaming at her Kind and Beautiful King to leave her, but he didn't, and he and the Midwife came at the last moment, catching the baby as it forced its way into the world.

'Turn on the light,' said The Midwife gently and the Princess closed her eyes. 'Look,' said The Midwife quietly.

'Oh, look at him,' said The Kind and Beautiful King.

The Princess didn't want to, but she saw that she had no choice.

She looked.

Looking right back at her was a beautiful baby. Tiny, with large dark blue eyes. the Princess allowed herself for a moment, a bit of hope. She studied him. She looked carefully for Cold Ice in his eyes, but she could only see a wise, old soul.

'You're like me,' she whispered to the baby and she allowed herself to touch him. The Midwife and The Kind and Beautiful King withdrew, and she touched her child and put her hand on his back and felt him breathe. She smelled his new little body.

He smelled just the same as The Kind and Beautiful King. She couldn't smell Monster or Danger or Snake. The little boy-baby studied his mother's face. He didn't make a sound. He waited patiently.

The Princess counted his ten little fingers and ten little toes and felt the whorl of his little ear.

She felt the fluff of hair on his little head and she wiped the blood from his little cheek.

Still, the little boy-baby looked calmly at his mother.

The Princess allowed herself to look at the rest of his body and she saw that she'd been so wrong to be afraid. She felt her heart grow and bloom with love and she fell hard and fast for the little boy that she held so tightly in her arms and she told him how sorry she was. the Princess sobbed and cried and covered his little face with kisses.

Exploring 'Beautiful Boy'

To: Sophie
From: Pat
The baby boy chapter made me feel very emotional. Your children have been very much a part of your healing journey. This baby boy will be so incredibly proud of you as you overcome this awful abuse and go out and speak on stage to others.

To: Pat
From: Sophie
That baby boy is the most amazing and gentle soul. He's very special and people seem drawn to his light.
I feel like it's coming to an end now.

As far as where I am in the therapy, I have more to do that I don't need or want to put in the book. I want to work on it for me only, with you, but I'm not sure how to as I think I need to be able to receive a handhold or touch if it gets too **much**.

~ Part Five ~

Rebuilding

let them come
images dark and now
let light follow
through cracks inside your soul
in, through and out they go
They are not welcome
here at my table
They have no seat
no food to eat
in, through and out they go.

Sophie Olson

The Mission and the Purpose

Spring

Pat and I began to have frequent discussions about self-publishing *The Flying Child*. I found myself torn between an excitement at taking this forward and an overwhelming fear of the consequences. I couldn't see how I could work in the field of survivor activism, publish my story, and stay anonymous and safe. My path to a life worth living was tantalisingly visible to me but felt frustratingly out of my reach and I knew it would be a fight to overcome these significant challenges. With the support and encouragement of Pat, I got through the days when my anxiety felt overwhelming and found the courage to show others my manuscript of *A Cautionary Fairy Tale for Adults*.

From day one I've been under no illusion that desire and drive would be enough and it is not as simple as one person starting a movement for change. I have met many survivor activists, all unique but working towards this collective goal. As Jon-Jay Needham* said to me recently, *this is about 'we' and 'us', not 'me' and 'I'* and how right he is.

Initially, collaboration came in the form of encouragement from others. Persistent networking and belligerent and dogged contacting of those whose work I admired, whose articles, podcasts, productions I related to. I began to share my manuscript with a wide range of people: journalists, producers, activists, charities and psychologists. One of the first people I shared it with was an acquaintance of mine, Kate Algar – a local artist. At the time I wanted illustrations in the book but felt she needed to read it to understand what I was looking for.

---

*Jon-Jay Needham is as a survivor and serving police officer working to improve services and make positive change for victims and survivors of CSA and sexual violence. He is an ambassador for The Survivors Trust.

I'm sharing it with my toes curled in embarrassment that she might see me as terribly self-absorbed and grandiose with a puffed sense of self-importance.

Time to let those conditioned patterns of thinking go. This is about helping others change and that begins with sharing your story with someone other than me.

I haven't actually sent it yet. She is expecting it though.

Good then send it off . . . you have to begin somewhere.

My anxiety is still really awful.

Ask yourself what you are anxious about. Is it because you are daring to tell people about it for the first time?

I don't think it is. I'm further away from achieving what I wanted than I was three weeks ago. I really don't think it is that. My story is the only thing that I feel hopeful about.

So, keep working with your story. Right now it is giving you a focus and stopping you from focusing on ill health. What about Barnardo's and NSPCC . . . what would they do with such a story to help prevent abuse?

Manuscript Replies

I had expected most people to ignore my request to read the fairy tale manuscript because why would they take time to read a story about such an 'unpalatable' subject, from a random stranger?! I did, however, receive a few responses and these were instrumental in what happened next, in particular the one from Kate. She was the first 'non survivor' acquaintance I had shared it with and waiting for her response had been nerve-wracking because I knew her. I had feared I might never hear from her again but was very encouraged by her response. It was the much-needed encouragement I needed to start letting this story go.

> **Just got some feedback from Kate who has started reading the book. Feels like a massive step!**
>
> Any response to feeling shocked, etc. or just commenting in general?
>
> **Good, I think! She has asked to read the extra chapters too so something about it must be capturing her interest, even if she doesn't feel she's the right artist for it.**
> **She then sent me another message saying it was playing on her mind. It's exactly what I want it to do. Play on people's minds.**

Kate wrote her initial review of the fairy tale.

> *I started to read your book last night. It's brilliant and horrific in equal measure. I don't know if my drawings are up to it, but I would love to have a go at creating something that I think fits your writing. For now, I'll keep on reading and thinking. It's incredibly powerful, Sophie. I can see how it would be commercial, niche and a vital tool all at the same time.*

I then received an email from a counsellor. She had been sent the manuscript with my permission by a survivor friend of mine.

I've had really positive feedback from a counsellor. It really encourages me to keep on fighting for this. I'll forward it to you . . .

Please thank your friend for letting me read her story. I was gripped from the beginning and sat to read the whole thing in one go. The psychological and mystical aspect of the tale is fascinating and really made me stop and think deeply about the events. For me, the use of character and symbolism actually made for a better understanding of the trauma than if this had been written in a standard biographical format. Importantly, the fantasy/escapism aspect also makes the piece accessible to any age of reader which is so crucial if changes are to be brought about.
It is hugely personal but so urgent and I thank her again for taking the time to write it down. I will be thinking about this for a long time to come.

My instinct was correct. *The Flying Child* was making people think. I saw for the first time the power of speaking out. I wanted to reach more people and I made a vow to myself that if anyone asked to read it, I would say yes. I was beginning to lose the shame that had kept me silent for so long, but unfortunately not all feedback was as encouraging as this. Survivor Activism is an effective people sifter. When you talk openly about CSA you quickly see the cracks appear in relationships that weren't as solid as they might have once seemed. I saw first-hand, the stigma of CSA. I lost a few people I cared about, and I'm not alone in my experience. Negative responses to disclosure are common and one of the biggest challenges we face. Of course, those who respond badly would never admit it to others. It would be like admitting you were secretly racist or hated women or kicked your dog. CSA experience should be a protected characteristic, and the behaviour I've observed is unacceptable on grounds of discrimination and hate. It is miserable to be on the receiving end of silencing and ignorant bigotry. Silence perpetuates abuse and the only people who truly benefit from it are the perpetrators.

* * *

I told my story to the NSPCC, working closely with a writer at their Real-Life story department. I was interviewed and my story written up and put on file, to be used when appropriate, with my permission, in the media. Later on, this did happen and it was strange to see my own story written in someone else's words. I am grateful to the charity for their respectful approach and careful handling of the process – I couldn't fault it – but I do find it interesting that since then I have seen a shift, and survivors themselves are taking on the role of educator, writer, trainer, consultant, and researcher. This is a healthy, empowering, and necessary shift. Survivors hold the key to sustainable change because we have an insight non-survivors, through no fault of their own, lack. It is a shift that not all will accept without resistance, as that would mean changing public perceptions of survivors as too vulnerable, fragile, or even mentally unwell to work on a level playing field as some who believe their degrees and time spent studying us, might make them better equipped to educate others *about* us.

Just told my story.

Well done. Make sure you are well grounded after telling the story.
How was the NSPCC and how did you feel telling the story and now afterwards? Your idea for the charity may be something you can grow as a dream in the background.

**I felt very much in control telling my story. I felt it was important, especially linking my background and class, and felt it would be beneficial for others to help raise awareness and educate. I spoke mostly about the psychological abuse as I believe that is the part of grooming that needs to be understood. I spoke less about the sexual abuse, as the word speaks for itself, but I told her that the abuse culminated in rape at the age of nine years old. That was a first for me.
Afterwards I felt OK. A bit detached, a bit anxious. I am struggling a lot with my pain levels, yesterday and today. They haven't been this bad for a while now.
And I felt astounded that I was telling this story, whilst he walks on this earth.**

Speaking on the phone and saying the word rape is a massive step forward considering your first reaction when I said the word to you for the first time. All these wonderful changes you have made! And yes, as you rightly say, he is walking the earth. Detachment is normal and part of coping with the reality and your pain shows it is related to anxiety. Try accepting that and negotiate with all your stiffness, tension, and pain. Its old stuff being revisited in the body.

I think I need to talk about this more with you face to face. Even now this conversation is hard. It's hard to read when you write the word. I think it must be because I know you. The person today was a stranger. It's an issue I need to overcome to be free of this. The body memory is intense and feels like it's in control of me.

Yes, I agree and that's why you need to be in a safe place to speak about your story before you take it further. Going further than that will need more practice. Body memories . . . work with your pushing away again as if you are pushing him further and further out of your life.

I can't do anything on my feet as I'm flat on my back because of the pain.

Nice belly breaths and mentally visualise extending your arms and chest for breath.

I had another response to the manuscript soon after this, from an audio producer, Redzi Bernard – another acquaintance at the time and someone I felt would be capable of creating something out of the fairy tale. She replied saying she wanted to pitch to BBC Radio 4. I was asked by survivor friends who knew of my plans if they could read the book and I asked Pat's opinion on this as I was concerned my story might trigger them.

> They must be the judge and you will be an incredible encouragement to them when they see how far you have come. It is always good to see those in front because it gives others the seeds to grow their own power to move forward.

Talk About
The Flying Child Project

My experience with the NSPCC and the responses I was receiving all supported the realisation that my story could be useful to others. The previous conversation with the professionally curious Head Teacher, Clare Brunet, swam back into focus, stimulating plans for a presentation to teachers that would later become The Flying Child Project, and I was keen to put them into action.

It was around this time I joined the Angles Network*: I received media training, met other survivors working in the field and for the first time identified that my own work was becoming a form of activism – that I was a survivor activist.

---

*Angles is a Heard (formally On Road Media) project that brings media influencers together with people with lived experience of sexual violence and domestic abuse, and/or who work in the sector, promoting new content and a better understanding of the issues.

The Power of Art

I decided I needed to do some more processing and decided to work on one of the earlier chapters: *All The Wrong Things.*

> **To: Sophie**
> **From: Pat**
> OK we can read this out loud next time. How did you feel as you were writing about his breathing? Next, you could illustrate the book with him in monster form, as the child would see him, so these disgusting noises start to be associated with him specifically.

> **To: Pat**
> **From: Sophie**
> I felt sick and anxious writing about it.
> I've sent another email with more, because it was another chapter that perhaps I needed to write out as it triggered quite a lot.

> **To: Sophie**
> **From: Pat**
> Thank you, Sophie. I will go through this tonight.

[See Picture Two – Bath]

> **To: Pat**
> **From: Sophie**
> This one has been difficult and set me back a bit. I'm finding it hard to get myself up today.

> **To: Sophie**
> **From: Pat**
> OK, I have a few mins now to get back to you . . . taking this large black figure . . . I want you to shrink him and put him into the bath, shivering and cold. Draw Sophie as the large figure instead. Then write down all the things you would like to say to him now . . . The feelings he has left you with, the triggers you experience, and

when you get tired of doing this, stop and breathe and leave it . . . come back and continue until the feelings are spent . . . if that makes sense.

To: Pat
From: Sophie
OK.

To: Sophie
From: Pat
Let me know how it goes and how it feels.

[See Picture Three – Shame]

To: Sophie
From: Pat
In your new picture you are now in control and have power. What do you want to say to the monster now?

To: Pat
From: Sophie
It felt hard and triggering. The sounds were clear in my head, as was the rest of it then.

To: Sophie
From: Pat
So, these sounds are important triggers, as we thought.

I would like to invite you to think about how powerful you are becoming with your story and the contacts you are making. How in your mind you are beginning to take back your power and diminishing his in such a skillful and empowering way. It's far more powerful than a court hearing could ever be and eventually his case will go to the world.

What would you like to say to him shivering in the bath? Do you want to see the book being read to him? . . .how would you see him on the receiving end of it all so that you can diminish the power he has over you?

To: Pat
From: Sophie
I'm not sure I can do that. This drawing has made me want to draw

more. Maybe I will be able to when I've drawn what's in my mind. It's the sounds that are triggering this.

To: Sophie
From: Pat
OK, go with the flow of what's happening.

To: Pat
From: Sophie
Why am I feeling so unsafe?

To: Sophie
From: Pat
Because you are daring to confront him instead of remaining silent and because you are now taking charge of what you would like to do with him and the situation.
    He looks much better in the bath!
    Perhaps down the plug hole even.

To: Pat
From: Sophie
I only feel like being shut away in my bedroom. Anywhere else makes me feel unsafe and out of control.

To: Pat
From: Sophie
This one has been triggered by sounds and writing the chapter 'All The Wrong Things'. The question is how to release myself from these snakes now.

[See Picture Four – Snakes]

To: Sophie
From: Pat
These drawings are amazing, and you don't need an illustrator for your book. These snakes now need to be given back to him where he is miserably sitting in his cold bath. These snakes belong with him and the sounds that went with them.

To: Sophie
From: Pat
Thanks. I'm working on it.
I don't think it should be the bath as the bath can be triggering too. Best to be an underground place. Another world.

To: Pat
From: Sophie
OK, wherever you would like to put them, along with him eventually . . . because he needs to be united with all of his gross stuff, forever.

[See Pictures 5 – The Pit]

To: Sophie
From: Pat
Wow, this is truly amazing. Your illustrations are sublime, and you could easily be a children's book illustrator. Such a truly talented person. I will be very upset if you ever harm those wrists and arms again. Look at the talents and the courage you possess. Nothing can hold you back, so reach for the stars.

To: Pat
From: Sophie
Thank you, I don't think I'm good enough for that though.

To: Sophie
From: Pat
I looked at everything in detail, including his watch! The more I look at that picture, the more powerful it becomes and the power the book has given you. People's stories are so important, and even more so when they are told to the world.

To: Pat
From: Sophie
With regards to harming behaviours, I just don't know if I'll ever be able to stop. Thank you for today's session. Sorry I said I felt flat. It lifted as I drove and sang! It is because harming is a hard topic to talk about, but I'm determined to conquer it.

To: Sophie
From: Pat
The harming was a coping mechanism – self-hatred and self-loathing become part of the narrative we tell ourselves and that is the lens we use to explain why we deserve to hurt . . . but it was never yours. It's the wrong narrative. Begin with gratitude.

To: Pat
From: Sophie
I would like to be able to do that. I'm never really still, partly because I'm physically uncomfortable a lot of the time but partly because I have this energy inside me. I've been thinking a lot about this anger too. How on earth to dispel it. Safely?

To: Sophie
From: Pat
So, keep channelling the anger. I am thinking if you draw a ladder thrown down to him you have accepted that you don't have enough anger and destruction in you to kill him. Anger is wonderful for motivation. It makes you write your book but if it gets out of hand it is like a Californian fire and then everything is burned to pieces. The anger now needs to be directed outwards to the many systems that failed you and still are failing others. If a 14-year-old can get up and start a movement for the planet, you can do the same for abuse.

To: Pat
From: Sophie
First of all, the book needs to be published.

To: Sophie
From: Pat
Then that is the focus.
My feeling is once it is broadcast, someone will help you take it forward. Finding your voice has been an important part of your recovery from all of this.

To: Pat
From: Sophie
Yes, me too, which is why I feel the audio documentary is important, but I also feel out of my depth and a bit lost with it too.

To: Sophie
From: Pat
So, calm it and focus on what you want to achieve. What do you want to really say and what changes do you want to make? Draw a nice powerful picture of Sophie taking her book to the world. Just as your picture took the power out of him . . . you now want to turn every disgusting thing he ever did to you into blossoms, and give them to the world. This shows that no matter how dark life gets, light always follows.

To: Pat
From: Sophie
Some things can't be undone. The physical toll it took on my body. I am so angry about that. I wasn't meant to be like this. I can't undo this. I know I can't. A lot of my anger is held in my body – in my spine.

Later . . .

I've got something else on my mind. The ladder. I haven't put it in my picture as I can't bring myself to do so but not giving him a ladder is making me feel uneasy. Sounds stupid probably.

That's fine re the ladder. You may not want to do it at all, or just not at the moment. Maybe he needs to own everyone's pain for a while.

I'm feeling murderous tonight. I want to kill him. I wish he was dead. I really wish he was dead.

Those feelings of extreme anger are signs for me that you are beginning to feel again.

Time to Create Change

One day, as a direct result of my step into the world of survivor activism, it occurred to me that I could simply stop fighting. It felt like my whole life had been a fight: a fight to survive, to hide. A fight to pretend, to forget, to die, to recover, to move on and to live. I had moments of positivity where I believed I'd mustered enough strength to start my life, but I would quickly become demoralised. Where and how would I start when life had carried on without me? I had no proper qualifications. It was too late to go back to university and I didn't really want to anyway. Once had been enough. My sewing and crochet business, that provided an income well below minimum wage, was taking a toll physically. I lived with a condition that made higher paid work impossible. I couldn't sit all day at a supermarket checkout. I couldn't continue with Montessori teaching – a job I'd done for a while until pain levels made me stop, but even if I could have physically managed these things, my confidence was impacted by the abuse and by the trauma of what had happened next. I had no courage or self-belief in myself to even try. I claimed benefits instead and I felt like my contribution to the world was useless. *A drain on society* had been the prediction of my university tutor and here I was fulfilling it.

And yet . . . I had a spark of rage inside me. A deep sense of injustice. All of this felt so unfair. I had a brain. I had started life with a healthy body and mind. I had been complete, and the Evil King had stolen parts of me. Whilst my contemporaries had been gaining degrees and experience in the workplace I had been trying to survive. I hated how someone like me was viewed by society. I hated how unfair it was that it was acceptable for me to say, *No, I don't work because I have depression, bipolar, a mental illness* BUT unacceptable for me to say, *I don't work because I am trying to survive Child Sexual Abuse.*

I began to wonder what it might feel like to stop *fighting* all the time and instead speak freely about abuse because it *was my lived experience.* Survival had been my education. I understood trauma, the impact on the child and adult, the stigma and the misunderstanding, and the lack of support, from a perspective impossible to gain from academic study. I also recognised how a better understanding of CSA and the consequences on the human mind, body and soul might result in a better outcome for the survivor. I tried to explain to Pat my thoughts around this and began with my frustration around (and alternative to) this idea of survivors feeling pressured to 'move on' and 'recover' from one of the most heinous and traumatising crimes imaginable.

The Flying Child

To: Pat
From: Sophie
I've had a lightbulb moment (I think).
    Here goes . . .
    The general idea behind traditional therapy/ treatment for sexual violence is that you process, in a safe environment, the traumatic memories, with the ultimate goal of 'moving on' and leaving it behind you, free to live your life, unburdened by the past events.
    Some survivors may be unable to feel that they can fully move on even after therapy but what if that's OK? What about the survivors who feel that the violation of the body affected their soul and that the abuse became part of them, the people who go through therapy and think, now what? Or worse, find themselves slipping back again, wondering if they need more therapy and if they can ever truly be free?
    What if these people are told that it's OK to not move on and leave it behind you? If you can't move on then don't, but change the way you view that. It's not that they've failed or are too damaged, but that they are choosing to use what happened to them instead, in a positive and powerful way.
    The gift of adversity in this case becomes their super-power, unique to survivors of abuse that can be used to raise awareness, influence change and help other survivors to find their voice.
    First-hand wisdom is invaluable as it evokes an emotional response from others which opens further doors, e.g. persuading people or organisations to donate money to fund further therapy for other survivors of abuse, research, or to influence a shift in behaviour, including how survivors are treated in society. It can also encourage other survivors to find their own voices (think of the #metoo movement) thereby creating an army of voices.
    Ultimately, any programme of therapy needs to lead to the opportunity to become part of a bigger network of voices, helping to influence a systemic change.
    So, I've run this concept of 'moving on' past [survivors] – women with different experiences of sexual violence and they are in total agreement. One views it as losing a part of her identity

by letting go entirely. Another describes the pressure to 'let go' but she can't – and feels that she's a burden if she keeps seeking help. One survivor described joining the support groups and 'finding people who spoke her language'.

I see my work as being with people and able to remove my mask and be myself. If I let go and move on then I lose that feeling, which I can't do, because I am that person who was abused. It did define me but I'm choosing to use that to my advantage now and work with it. This empowers me more than medication ever has.

To: Sophie
From: Pat
Making lots of sense and as you continue working with this, eventually the identity of 'I am an abused person' falls away and it becomes 'I am a person helping others through abuse'. Some may want to keep the identity all their lives because they don't know who they are without it or how else to explain their struggle on the mainland. We will take a look at this tomorrow once we have dealt with any other business.

To: Pat
From: Sophie
Yes, but I'm looking at it differently. What if there's a third option? When deciding to not let go but to view it differently, not as illness, not as a struggle, but with absolute acceptance, after it has been processed in a safe way, with specialist and intensive therapy.

Survivors of CSA often feel isolated. The struggle on 'the mainland' is a result of the shame, stigma, silence and unpalatability of sexual violence. The more we are able to speak our stories, the more we help reduce this in society as a whole. The easier life on the mainland becomes.

If I'm OK with my identity being a person with lived experience, who can now use these experiences to help others, then does that identity need to fall away? I don't think it does. If it's a problem and it keeps me in perpetual victim mode, then it's unhealthy, but I don't feel like a victim anymore. I did before, especially when I was attending appointments for my mental health. The victim feeling has gone away now, and I know it's never coming back. I will always be a victim of a crime, but I don't need to be a victim for the rest of my life because my mindset has changed. I will always be a survivor though, and there are consequences to that. That's normal and I will no longer be ashamed of my normal responses to trauma.

~ Part Six ~

Consolidation

What the Doctors Didn't See

Summer

[See Picture 6 – Brace]

> **To: Pat**
> **From: Sophie**
> Hi Pat,
>   I've done this picture for a blog post about body memories but I wanted to share the picture with you as part of our work.

> **To: Sophie**
> **From: Pat**
> OK, that looks amazing. Will talk soon.

> **To: Pat**
> **From: Sophie**
> **I have more pictures I wanted to share with you.**

[See Pictures 7–12]

> **To: Pat**
> **From: Sophie**
> I knew there was a reason for these pictures I drew in 2009!

> **To: Sophie**
> **From: Pat**
> You drew them in 2009! Wow, all that time ago and you couldn't talk about them. Where were you at that time when you were drawing this?

To: Pat
From: Sophie
In the psychiatric hospital. I didn't put the words on them though. I've just added those today.

To: Sophie
From: Pat
Did you want to put words then or you couldn't?

To: Pat
From: Sophie
I couldn't.

To: Sophie
From: Pat
But no one asked you about your drawings?

To: Pat
From: Sophie
The psychiatrist said they were very interesting.
    But continued to treat me with more medication.
    It's all I could do in group therapy sessions. Other people made notes and I did this. Not for anyone else to see and I don't know where they came from at the time. Now I think they're very relevant.

To: Sophie
From: Pat
Yes, they are. I can't believe that no one asked you what they were about.

To: Pat
From: Sophie
I also made them out of clay.

To: Sophie
From: Pat
Oh, my goodness, how powerful is that?

To: Pat
From: Sophie
He gave me more labels and then told me the words that stuck with me for years.

'You have a severe and enduring mental illness. You will never live without medication and will always need support.'

To: Sophie
From: Pat
I can never understand why you would say that to a patient even if you thought it.

To: Sophie
From: Pat
Yes, it is pompous. He was arrogant and he became frustrated with me. I wasn't getting better, yet I also challenged his opinions, which he didn't like. I didn't fit nicely into any box, that was the problem.

I shared details with Pat of who the psychiatrist was and the books he'd published, and I described how triggered I'd felt when I met this man at my first appointment in 2009. He was a similar 'type' to the Evil King. He spoke with the same public school education accent. He wore similar clothes, had the same body type, eye colour, demeanour and confidence. I started that appointment triggered, with a sense of being at the wrong end of an enormous power imbalance, and most definitely on the back foot.

> A client has found great comfort in your new blog as her poor body is racked by body memories.

> **She's not alone. Body memories are the worst legacy of sexual violence because it feels like you have no control over them. Like I said in the post, it's about learning how to live with them and tackling each one. I know I still have the basement one to tackle and I still don't know how. I have to, though, because it worked well for my 'Summertime' chapter, and I want the same release from these memories too.**

They will come when the time is right and you have to 'know' that you can trust what the body memories are telling you. Sometimes the body memories are more accurate than mind memories because they don't contain constructs of what might be happening . . . They relay back what did happen.

I'm not sure how you ever trust the body memories on their own. Even the most fragmented memories were memories – but to have just a blank seems so much harder.

Body memories, though fragmented, need to be spoken to in the same way as the inner child. Talking to the memories . . . 'What are you trying to tell me? What was going on to you at this time? What were you feeling?' They too will tell their story . . . Once upon a time there was a little girl's body . . .

It's not something I can do myself. It makes me feel so unsafe. I need to do it with you.

That's fine, we can do that.

But what if I still don't get anywhere?

I think you instinctively already know what these memories are about . . . by virtue of where they are most felt in your body.

I'm not sure I do. It's vocalising that's always been the key for me. If I can't identify the cause and articulate it, then I remain stuck in fear.

That's fine, we can find a time to vocalise it. The key lies in your 'interesting' pictures and labels you have now attached to it.

Lots of them had their arms over their heads. Like this one. It makes me laugh as I was supposed to be writing notes from a bloody useless CBT lecture but got distracted by drawing these instead!

Your drawings are far more profound than CBT! Was this connected with the abuse or did these occur afterwards?

Also, I can't read the words around the group of people. What was going on for you at the time of all of this?

It was all connected with abuse. I knew what had happened to me, but I was silent and kept pushing it away. I went to these groups because I was going through the motions of engaging with the treatment in [the hospital] but I was absolutely desperate inside. These drawings became my focus. In art therapy, I made them out of clay. I felt misunderstood and just wanted to die. I tried to kill myself whilst at the hospital but that just made the misunderstanding even worse. It was a terrible time, and I didn't care for anything or anyone or myself. It was the worst possible place for me at that time.

Did the psychiatrist never ask what the pictures were about?

Actually, he may have done. I was too shut down though.

But you might have wondered seeing that and encouraged the art much more.

Yes. If only I had had that opportunity. I was writing constantly at the time as well.
The art therapy was terrible. The therapist was disinterested in the work produced and because of this, it felt like an unsafe group for me. Art therapy gives people the opportunity to release deep trauma but there was no one to contain that or support us. I would go back to my room and find innovative ways to self-harm, to cope with the feelings it brought up. Most of this went unnoticed, which suited me perfectly as I felt deep shame about my harming. There was one amazing nurse who did have more insight and she saved my life when I collapsed one night, but I wished she hadn't because the consequences of that were punitive and will stay with me forever.

But now you can't possibly feel that your life being saved wasn't or isn't worthwhile? You are now helping to save one of my client's life because she knows out there in the universe is a person who has experienced the same and survived.

No, I don't feel that anymore.
Looking back over the pictures it's like I was drawing my future. I didn't know I'd have more children at that stage . . . and the 'helping' one never made any sense to me. I wasn't involved with groups of women and didn't feel any connection with anyone else like I did when I joined your groups.
I do wonder what the arm over the head is about though.
And the ones with the large man. I remember drawing these and that it was myself as an adult in an adult relationship I was in around that time but when I'd finished, I looked back at it and realised that the proportions were wrong, and I had drawn myself as child-sized. It was like my own brain had tricked me into looking right at something that I'd got so good at pushing away. I remember the shock I felt then.

* * *

Do you know what the drug haloperidol is?

As far as I remember it is a strong sedative used to quieten down psychotic episodes. Why?

When I was in [the psychiatric hospital] I trusted an EMDR specialist. He pushed and pushed me to tell him the most graphic memories of the abuse. It went on for ages and at the end, I saw his erection under his trousers, and I realised that he was sexually aroused — by my words describing Child Sexual Abuse. I decided at that moment that there was just no point. I was already an inpatient. What was the fucking point anymore if even the so-called experts are the same. I tried to kill myself at the hospital and it was because of that doctor, who had made me trust him. My distress and suicidal intention were treated with haloperidol. Forcibly injected into me with the most terrible side effects.

Oh my god . . . it is an extremely powerful drug and more so when injected. Sophie, how horrendous for you. Sadly, it does not totally surprise me. It is important for the 'experts' themselves to be monitored and supervised and to have a space to process and release, so they can retain some normality to their lives.

My experiences in [the hospital] – some were awful like I just described, yet it also kept me alive.

Chapter 35

Severe and Enduring

'But I don't want to go among mad people,' Alice remarked.
'Oh, you can't help that,' said the Cat, 'we're all mad here. I'm mad. You're mad.'
'How do you know I'm mad?' said Alice.
'You must be,' said the Cat, 'or you wouldn't have come here.'

– Alice in Wonderland, Lewis Carrol

On the day her daughter turned nine, the Princess finally went Mad. Or so she was told.

The Big Black Door had remained firmly shut, locked, and bolted for many years and the Princess lived her life but the effort of keeping it shut and bolted grew harder and harder every day until it weighed heavily upon her heart and soul and her mind began to crack.

As her Captured Mind cracked, the photographs began to find a way out. They rolled into a tight spiral and pushed through the keyhole, and they slid out from the gap under the door and the crack in the hinge and the Princess awoke every morning to find a new one had landed on her in the night, and she couldn't help but see it. Then, when she looked in the mirror to put on her make-up, she saw there were photographs stuck to the glass and she ripped them off, but staring right back at her was the Evil King. So, she stopped putting on make-up and she stopped looking in mirrors.

One day, the Princess took her children for a walk in the woods and as she watched them climb in the trees, she saw the photographs of Shitting in the Woods Day had pinned themselves to their colourful coats. Another day, when she was walking in The World with her beautiful boy, a large photograph at the top of the escalator caught her eye so they had to take the stairs instead.

When she tried to go to The Kind and Beautiful King for comfort, he put his beautiful arms around her and kissed her gently, but the Princess felt hard, soft Snakes and tasted the saltiness of a monstrous tongue, and she began to shrink, and The Kind and Beautiful King was sad. the Princess cried to see him so sad but there was nothing she could do.

The Princess began to despair.

'My Big Black Door is useless!' she cried, and she didn't know what to do. On the eve of her daughter's ninth birthday, the Princess went to her bedroom to give her a kiss goodnight and she saw, to her horror, picture after picture. They were on the bed, on the walls and on the floor and as she looked in Fear at her daughter, she could only see her own nine-year-old self, looking back at her, wrapped in a million writhing Snakes. So, the next day, she lost her mind. Or so they said.

She couldn't say what was wrong as she hadn't learned how to speak the words and she didn't want to. She wanted to shut the Big Black Door and seal it properly, once and for all, and never think of it again.

'Take this pill' said The Doctors, in the hospital in which they had hidden the Princess. 'It will balance your mind.'

So, the Princess did as she was told, as she had always done, but it didn't work. Still her mind continued to crack.

'Try this one too,' said The Doctors, waiting for her to swallow her pills and they added more and more until the Princess could hear them rattling inside her Body.

A pill to sleep, a pill to quieten her mind, a pill to make her see colour, a pill to make sure that the colour wasn't too bright, a pill to wake up, a pill to stop the sickness caused by all the pills, and on and on it went and none of them worked. Until one day, the Princess said, 'No more!' and she refused to take any at all.

'But you are mad,' said The Doctors. 'You are ill. You have lost your mind. You must take the pills.'

But the Princess refused because she knew deep down, she wasn't Mad. She knew her mind was captured, and her soul had been stolen, and she needed help to shut the Big Black Door once and for all, and she needed to find the words to explain, so she tried, and she tried but she wasn't ready. The words were too big and stuck too far down to be spoken and although she managed to speak, the words were mixed up and made no sense to The Doctors. She stuttered and cried and raged and begged and her words fell out, upside down and inside out. The Doctors didn't understand tales of Snakes and Shadows and Cold Ice and Cages. They told her firmly once more that she was quite Mad and that her Madness was Severe and Enduring and that she'd never be well. Then they made her lie on a bed and they forced the medicine into her Body instead, with a sharp needle that pierced through her hip and the Princess roared with rage and frustration.

'There, there,' they said, and backed away.

You need to get out of here, whispered the Old Witch from within, as the Princess slipped into a deep sleep.

*Exploring
'Severe and Enduring'*

> How long was your stay in the hospital?

I was in rehab (for addiction) for 28 days but I ended up staying there and was transferred to the general programme, so 4 months inpatient stay in total.

> And during that period of time how much time was devoted to therapy or any other form of holistic therapy?

In the addiction programme, it was very intense therapy all day and followed by 12 step meetings during the evening. All compulsory.
In the general programme there was a [therapy] programme, but it was non-compulsory. Some holistic e.g. art, Pilates, yoga, was offered. Not much though and nothing at the weekend, although I think they brought in organised walks after I left.

> What sort of intense therapy . . . 1:1 with a psychiatrist? What else was included?

It's hard to remember exactly but it was disappointingly infrequent in the general programme. Perhaps once/twice a week we saw a consultant. Therapist one to one varies depending on urgency, I think.
Holistic therapy, just yoga, Pilates, art, but not really therapy as such. I think this varies between different hospitals. NHS. Private. Private and NHS patients are mixed together at [that hospital].
In the general programme, a lot of people didn't engage at all and sat in front of the tv or stayed in their rooms. Lots were too drugged to engage.
In the rehab programme every bit of time was used, and it was intense too, so along the right lines, but, as you know, such an inappropriate environment for a vulnerable woman

and I wasn't able to talk about my trauma. In my small group of people there were male sex addicts. I was encouraged to form strong bonds with them, but I was disgusted by them. But I can understand the thinking behind the addiction treatment programme, and it probably works if that's the reason you're there. It just was wrong for me. And it was too punitive in its approach which I found infantilising. I never felt empowered to take responsibility for myself.

In some cases, addiction is a coping mechanism for underlying trauma and therefore the programme is a sticking plaster. Trauma survivors need their deep wounds to be cleaned and sutured and the application of a large bandage that needs cleaning and changing daily. Without that, relapse is highly likely.

Yes, you're probably right. They believed that's what they were doing though. Maybe they did for some, if the deep wound wasn't too complex. Writing this chapter has had a physical effect on me. My heart races a bit.
I'm in a lot of physical pain today. Sitting at the computer hurts my back. I've written all of it on my phone for that reason, but I need a computer to edit. These are the days I need to watch because physical pain brings me down.

Ease the pain. Remember you have a new purpose now and you have already been told your book is powerful and it is . . . in many ways it is more chilling than presenting it as the 'real' story.
It's the first time I've read it myself with such concentration. It's a bit disconcerting.
I'm going to The Kingdom Of His today.

Take it very easy.

I wonder if I will find it hard to look at my family today.

You might but remember you have nothing to be guilty about.

* * *

I have let my husband read my story. It suddenly felt like the right time to do so. He reacted perfectly. Not too much sympathy although I can see that he's upset, and he said he cried all the way through.

This is amazing news. I am so pleased you have finally shared this with him. He will have a deeper understanding now of what you have been grappling to come to terms with all your life. For me your chapter of your descent into darkness is the most powerful explanation of flashbacks I have ever read, as you build up the camera pictures in your head and suddenly you let them go all at once. Your descriptions will hopefully bring a new understanding to the world of psychiatry and that is why true healing can never come about by medication. By sharing this with him you have, once again, had your story validated by someone you love and trust and the more you validate and the more validation you receive, the more you will realise that it is not you who is mad, but the monster you grew up with. He belongs in an institution for the criminally insane.

When we discover our purpose, it is difficult sometimes for the horse not to go from a trot into a gallop too quickly. We run the danger of becoming burned out. It is vital at this point to take care of the body and rest properly in the stable with comfortable bedding, good hay to eat, safety and security and especially loving kindness.

Intergenerational Trauma

I'm interested in the legacy of trauma and how it impacts the next generation too. Today has been a case in point. One of my children is struggling with how my poor mental health has made them feel. I think it's happening now because they see I might be stronger but don't believe I can be. It all comes under 'repercussions'. There is no genetic depression that runs through my family as far as I know. This is all a consequence of what happened to me. It threw me spinning out of orbit for the rest of my life and the legacy infected my children. But even deeper than that, genetically, how are they affected by this stuff? The studies on survivors of the holocaust talk about transgenerational trauma.

Everyone carries ancestral trauma so it's something that can't be avoided. It is part of the human condition. It's how we resolve it that's important. They are now watching you resolve it, and they have seen what happens if you don't.

Bearing Witness

We must all bear witness to other people's stories, so that we may act on preventing abuse from happening in the future.

This was a quote in an email response to the manuscript from the activist Purnima Govindarajulu and it encouraged the shift in my thinking from 'my story happened to me' to 'my story can be used to help others'.

I first read about Purnima, a Canadian woman of Indian origin, in a BBC news article describing her lobbying for a change in the law so adult survivors in India can report Child Sexual Abuse. I read about her upbringing, her abuse by a family member between the ages of 6 and 13, and the silence surrounding this abuse, hidden from her family under complex layers of shame, stigma, confusion, and reputation.

I felt an immediate connection to her and that I needed to make contact. I messaged her, not expecting to receive a reply but weeks later, an email arrived, apologising for the delay. She wasn't perturbed by this stranger contacting her out of the blue, she welcomed it and was keen to hear my story too.

After reading my manuscript she messaged again, asking if we could speak on the phone, so one day, late in the evening for her and early in the morning for me, we chatted, and it felt as easy as speaking to an old friend.

Purnima described relating to my story in a visceral way – in her words – *The flying out of my body, the demon sucking colours out of me and the world around me, freezing the words so they were stillborn before they left my mouth . . . Then as a survivor pretending in the world, I went from the timid please-everyone mask to the strong, independent competent mask.*

And she said those words to me about *'bearing witness'*.

I will forever be thankful to Purnima. She was one of the first survivor activists I met who was striving for change and actually doing something to influence it. I admire her strength. I used this shift in my thinking to shape plans that then began to come to fruition. All activists stand on the shoulders of giants and we take courage from those who have spoken before. My hope is that my activism and voice will bring a similar strength of spirit. I shared Purnima's response with Pat.

> There you go . . . we must just wait for the right time, and it will all happen without fear or shouting or demonstrations.

To: Pat
From: Sophie
Subject: Self-injury
Dear Pat.
 I've decided to try and write out the self-harming. It's not easy to write about but as I've had so much success with writing out the rest, I'm going to give it a go for this too. Please can you let me know what you think and what I could do next, to follow on from this?
 And after reading it, tell me honestly if you still think I can really recover. Did you know how badly I hurt/ have hurt myself in the past? I wonder if you might have turned me away if you'd realised it when we started the therapy.

Chapter 36

The Angry

'Perhaps the greatest risk any of us will ever take is to be seen as we really are.'

Cinderella, (2015)

The Princess's Angry heart was pounding inside her chest. Like a pot that had boiled over, she hissed and spat as she fought with her Kind and Beautiful King.

There was too much Anger inside her and it poured out like poison from an infected wound.

As it flowed, it was replenished by more; it was never ending. Anger had been hiding in her body, entwined with the twisted vertebrae, inside throbbing kidneys, lying dormant in veins and arteries and inside her heart. She was so angry at The World *and* the Shadow of Rocks *and* the Grey *and* the Evil King *and* now her Kind and Beautiful King, that she didn't know what to do with it and feared her heart may explode into a million pieces *and that she would die from it.*

Stop! screamed the Old Witch inside the Princess's head. *Stop!*

And the Princess, in her red mist, took herself as far away as she could, to stop, in the only way she knew how.

The Princess gasped with the pain of it as she attacked her own self, and the air that rushed into her angry lungs quelled the flames of rage, but it wasn't enough.

Anger rose again and surged through her Body and along her arm and into each finger, and she did it again. And again, and again, and again, until finally The Anger retreated in fear and the Princess could breathe again.

She sat calmly in a sea of red and surveyed the damage on her Body. Her skin cried and the Princess did nothing to comfort it. *Drip, drip, drip,* went the blood tears, and the Princess was glad. *You deserve it,* she thought, but the Old Witch grieved from deep within and the Princess was frightened.

She begged for death, but she feared it too.

The Old Witch whispered in her ear, *But what if?*

But maybe...

And simply, *Just wait.*

So, the Princess did. She waited for just a bit longer, just in case, because just maybe, and what if.

And The World carried on.

Exploring 'The Angry'

Thank you for being so honest. You have finally talked about something you feel so ashamed of... it is out and being talked about by you. It is flowing now and will do until it is finally released.
Would I have turned you away... probably not. If you had presented with violent or dangerous behaviour towards me as your therapist, then I would not have been able to work with you.
One day, Sophie, as you get deeper into your work, you may need to share this. There is no shame in what you tried to do because you couldn't escape. In spite of everything you are still here, and gradually you are freeing yourself of this wretched past. There will come a time soon where you will never want to do this again.

It has always been and continues to be my choice to do these things, although it never feels like a choice at the time. It's desperation to escape from the way I'm feeling at that moment.
I wrote these things to try and explain to you how bad this can be as it occurred to me on Saturday that even though you know my story, you can't fully understand this side of me if I don't tell you and therefore you can't help. I want to get help and to stop. I'm not actively suicidal and I'm not currently doing these things apart from the self-harm but that's occasional and not regular. It's not as severe as it is in that writing. But I have done these things a lot over the last 15 years or so and unfortunately it's never very far away. When I talk about slipping back, this is what I'm frightened of.
There has never been psychosis.

And I have never felt there was psychosis, only a desperate attempt to make sense of what had happened to you. Anger seems to be the dominant feature of this behaviour and when you are ready, I would like you to explore anger from the child's point of view. Who and what was she really angry about?

Did you know it was this bad?

Rather than how bad you are, I am more surprised that you are alive. So, with that in mind, the question arises as to why you would continue with the death plan because after a while death plans become futile and one can only then decide to live. And when one makes that decision, then anything is possible.

Yes, and I can honestly say that I don't have the death plan now, but something must change to stop me going back to it.

I would like, if possible, for you to illustrate your anger . . . drawing in colour can be very helpful in letting go. Then afterwards, do something practical, or go for a walk or cycle to let more of it go. This anger is locked in your cells, so work with the exercises I showed you for releasing anger.

I'm feeling so angry at the moment. Right now, I'm sitting where he abused me in the chapter called 'Campervan and Saxophone'.

Feel where the anger is in your body. Think about what you would want to scream at him and do to him at that time. You may need screaming time in your car . . . it really helps to park up and just let it go and let the words pour out as well. Anger is good at this stage, not at you but him. You did nothing wrong, and you could do nothing. You were a child trapped with a monster, but now you are the adult, and he is getting old and frail and he might think you too are frail and frightened, but you are not.
I have been waiting for this to come for a long, long time and your anger is completely justified.
It must be hard for you to go back [to the family home] and have the words for what happened to you there . . . like a holocaust survivor returning to Auschwitz. You have been on such a journey you should be so, so proud of yourself . . . you survived . . . you are profoundly talented and now you have something to live for . . . no fear. Tell the world what Auschwitz felt like in a beautiful middle-class home. The stereotype is that abusive acts only happen in poor families. We know

that's not true. Know that you can help prevent this from happening to other kids. Just prepare yourself mentally and physically . . . strengthen every bone in your body and go out there and deliver it to every organisation and every law court across the land.

Being able to speak openly to Pat about self-injury was such a relief after decades of silence. I knew that finding an alternative way of controlling any negative emotion was one of the biggest challenges I faced. When you've relied upon something to survive, changing the behaviour is not easy. It's like deciding not to eat when you feel hungry. Not to drink when you feel thirst. Not to respond to a change in weather with an extra sweater. Not to comfort yourself when feeling sad with a cosy blanket, Netflix, and a cup of tea.

At this point in therapy, I was preparing to record the documentary with Redzi as her latest pitch had been successful. It was going to be broadcast on BBC Radio Four and called 'The Last Taboo'.

I am being recorded for The Last Taboo tomorrow. It's going to be more of an interview now. I'm worried I won't be able to speak and articulate adequately. I have so much that I want to say but as you know the words sometimes get stuck.

Why don't you make bullet points of the most important things you want to say, almost like a mini script, so that you at least have some words to voice the ones that are difficult . . . and don't forget afterwards to tell yourself how amazing you are and how far you have come from that young woman who showed me a mask full of bricks! You are a very different person now!

Yes, I will. I've written lots of notes but condensing it into bullet points is a good idea. I will tell myself I'm amazing if I do a good job!

You can tell yourself you are amazing anyway because you are not wearing a brick mask!

No! Definitely not wearing that anymore!!

* * *

How did your recording go?

It went well. Redzi was very happy with it and described me as articulate, said that I spoke clearly and with visual language, making it easy for others to imagine some of what I'd gone through.
And that it would be very hard to cut down as a lot of it was powerful and important.
She has until February/March now so we can revisit it and record more.

Chapter 37

The Journey

Poor little Snow White was very frightened alone in the woods. Darkness was falling and although she was not in the thickest part of the wood, she was still lost, lonely and afraid.

– Snow White, The Brothers Grimm

Although she had made her way out of the prison and away from The Doctors, the Princess was never far away from the now half-open Big Black Door. She knew she must do better at pretending so she put on her Mask of Bricks and made a vow *never* to remove it.

But the Mask of Bricks was heavy and it made her tired, and one day the Princess became so tired of life in The World that she tried to leave it.

She tried to spill her blood, but it would dry up and stop flowing.

She climbed to the top of a highest mountain and tried to jump into the sky, but the wind caught her and blew her back.

She tried to swallow poison, but it always turned to water.

'Why can't I leave The World?' she said in despair. 'I'm broken, I'm half-dead and I hurt all over. I will never grow tall and strong; I am crooked and bent. Why am I not allowed to leave?'

She felt an itch on her shoulder blade and reached behind her and felt in surprise the nub of a tiny wing. She had forgotten about the wings and felt the stirring of excitement quickly followed by Fear. She was afraid to feel excitement. What if they withered and died?

The tiny nub unfurled, and the little wing fluttered, giving her the strength to carry on for a little while longer.

The Princess and her wing decided they would go on a journey to see if they could find the way to mend her broken Body and release her Captured Mind.

This journey was difficult. Dragging the heavy Shadow of Rocks behind her, the Princess walked and walked through a dense forest. She was tired. The road was bumpy and steep and there were Traps and Tricks along the way.

She walked through a clearing and saw beyond her a beautiful sparkling lake. Its dazzling brightness intrigued the weary Princess and she moved closer, to read a sign nailed onto the slimy trunk of a sad-looking tree. The sign read,

> *Welcome to the lake of wine.*
> *Full immersion in this lake will make you forget dark Shadows and crawling Snakes. It will chase away your pains and it will wash away your Shame. You will emerge clean and joyous.*

The Princess stumbled in her eagerness to swim in the lake – and in she fell, headfirst.

As she swam, she found to her astonishment that the pains in her bent and twisted Body did indeed subside.

'How wonderful,' said the Princess.

She swam some more, and the Shadow of Rocks began to dissolve in the wine. the Princess's Body felt lithe and young as it moved gracefully through the silky liquid and when she looked inside her mind, pushing tentatively at the Big Black Door, like a tongue pressing at a throbbing tooth, she found that it didn't hurt so much.

'It's a miracle!' the Princess tried to say, but as she opened her mouth, the wine flowed in and down to her stomach. It poured into her lungs and through her veins. The more it filled up the Princess, the heavier she became, and she started to sink down, down, down, deeper and deeper until she feared she would be drowned at the bottom.

Help me, thought the Princess, and the little wing, hearing her thought, turned into a little fin and swam furiously. Slowly, slowly, the Princess began to rise from the murky depths, up and up towards the light sky above, until she emerged, choking and shivering, still bent and twisted, hurting even more than before, and dragging a larger, heavier Shadow of Rocks behind her.

The Princess saw it had been a Cruel Trick and she carried on with her journey.

By and by, the Princess came to another clearing, and nailed to the trunk of a dead-looking tree covered in thorns was a second sign. It read,

> *Magic Swords guaranteed to cut away Shadows once and for all in just one swipe.*

The Princess remembered the punishments she would inflict on her Useless Body and how good it felt to punish it.

She hated her Shadow of Rocks. It attached itself in places all over her Body and made those places infected and dirty. She wanted more than anything to get rid of it once and for all, so she looked carefully at the row of swords that stuck out of the muddy, brown earth. She chose one of the smallest swords. It was gold-coloured with a sharp, vicious-looking blade. the Princess took hold of it in both hands, lifted it high above her head and with a deep breath sliced the sword through the air, aiming at the dark Shadow of Rocks.

Instead of severing the Shadow as promised, the sword landed on her delicate Princess skin with a cruel thud, cutting bluntly through her tender flesh. Blood fountained and the Princess screamed in frustration and pain.

She selected a second sword. This one had sharp serrated teeth and the blade flashed as she swiped it through the air. Again, it didn't touch the Shadow, but ripped jaggedly through sinew and flesh. the Princess felt as if she were on fire. In a furious rage, the Princess grabbed all the swords and cut and hacked and sliced at the Shadow of Rocks, but it was too clever, sliding effortlessly out of the way every time. the Princess was so angry that she hacked and sliced and cut her Body over and over again, trying to cut away the dirty, infected places, until, wet with blood, the exhausted Princess fell to her knees. In utter despair, the Princess looked for something to cover the terrible wounds and to slow the fountains of blood but the only thing she could see was the Shadow of Rocks. She wrapped herself up in it and dragged herself on.

'You win,' she said, and the Shadow smirked and the Evil King, far, far away, heard and smiled.

The Princess limped on. She stopped at another sign. the Princess rubbed her weary eyes and read,

> *Eat your worries away in The Garden of Food! Destroy your shadows from the inside out!*

The Princess walked into a garden of food, and she was tempted by delicious cakes, freshly baked loaves, and plump, juicy fruit. They grew in abundance, weighing down the branches with their promises.

The Princess ate and ate and swallowed more and more and more in the hope that the food would consume the Shadow of Rocks as promised, but instead, a great sickness overcame the Princess and she vomited white maggots and bile.

Chapter 38

The White Witch and the Blossom Tree

In the old tales, kindness is the purest form of heroism. Find the character who meets the world with a big heart and an open hand, and you have found your hero or heroine.

– *Far Far Away*, Tom McNeal

The Princess was dying. Her breath came in ragged, shallow gasps and her vision was obscured by the black death that was creeping over her near-dead eyes.

'I can't do any more,' said the Princess, and she sat down next to a great tree and waited to die.

She stared at the tree. It was tall and magnificent and alive, covered in beautiful pale pink blossom that gently rained down from the branches, covering the Princess in its fragrant beauty. She noticed a small yellow door in the trunk of the tree and wondered who lived there.

She could see a sign on the door, and she struggled to make out the words that moved and blurred before her eyes.

It said,

Help Offered – for Frozen Statues, half-dead princesses, and Captured Minds. Masks not required.

That's me, thought the Princess. But she was worried it could be another Trick.

You have nothing more to lose, said the wing.

Searching in her mind for a bit of courage, the Princess secured her Mask of Bricks firmly on her face, stepped through the little door and went inside the beautiful, big blossom tree.

Inside, stood a White Witch.

'Welcome to the beginning of the end of your journey,' she said.

The Princess was distrustful. She watched the White Witch carefully and studied her face for signs of a Mask.

'You can come closer if you like,' said the White Witch but the Princess stayed back. She didn't trust the White Witch. the Princess asked the White Witch if she'd seen Snakes and Shadows.

'Yes,' said the White Witch, 'and I know how to help.'

The Princess thought it unlikely because if you know Snakes and Shadows, then you know that they are undefeatable.

The White Witch heard the Princesse's wonderings.

'In Time' she said and the Princess wondered if she was a fool.

The door opened and in walked a beautiful Princess, followed by four more. The White Witch reminded them gently that in lesson one, Masks were not required and, reluctantly, one by one, they removed their Masks and placed them on the table. There in front of the Princess stood a sorry collection of half-dead Princesses and Frozen Statues. Some dragged Shadows behind them. Some were bent and twisted. Some had lost parts of their minds. Some had parts of their bodies that had withered and died. They were burned and scarred. One opened her mouth to speak and the Princess saw that she couldn't. Her tongue had been partially cut out and it flopped uselessly against her chin.

The Princess could see that one had eaten so much in the garden of food that she had grown as large as a giant and could barely fit her bulky body through the door.

Another had eaten so little that she had no fat at all. Her bones clacked and clattered together as she walked, and the Princess could see straight through her transparent bony body. She wondered about the Trick of which she had fallen foul.

One had punished her Useless and Weak body so much that the Princess could see right through the holes and cuts in her Body to the room behind. She trailed drops of blood, and the

Princess wondered which bits of herself she had tried to cut out.

One was dripping wet from the lake of wine, and it dribbled out of her ears and mouth and eyes and dripped from the tendrils of her hair, leaving a puddle on the floor.

The Princess looked curiously at the Masks on the table.

There was a smiling, happy Mask, a joking and play-the-clown Mask, a timid, please-everyone Mask, a strong and competent Mask, and a perfect-in-all ways Mask.

Trust her, said the Old Witch quietly from within.

I have nothing more to lose, thought the nearly dead Princess and she too removed her Mask of Bricks and put it on the table with the others.

What can I say to this, Sophie? You have been to hell and back . . . you have experienced every kind of torture there is to experience, but you are still here and what's more, you want to help others. You are a very rare princess, and it is time for you to live. You will become increasingly stronger and you will never be seen as weak again. You are truly amazing. Your story has brought tears to my eyes at times. I do not know how you have survived but you have. This cannot happen without a phenomenal mind and strength beyond belief.

Thank you. I'm writing it but feel detached from it. I have a lot of work to do. I need to remember it all. It's not to torture myself. It is to kill it once and for all. I need to see clearly what I'm fighting so that nothing is left behind to catch me unawares.

Well, you have remembered a lot through your story, and you have remembered where you took yourself when your mind didn't want to be attached anymore. This does not happen lightly to someone as a child. It is not usual for a child to choose to check out from a really young age, unless it is something extremely horrific.

I'm frightened I'm never going to be free of it. Of him. My writing is a form of exorcism, but I'm frightened it's not enough. I feel like a fraud. When you tell me my story should be published, a voice tells me that I'll fail. You use words like rare and amazing and strong, but my mind is captured so I can't really think that of myself because he won't allow me to. I don't know yet if there is a happily ever after in this story.
Good night, white witch. Whilst my trust wasn't instant, I do trust you now, implicitly, and I certainly don't think you're a fool!

Chapter 39

The Women and the Purpose

Just living is not enough . . . one must have sunshine, freedom, and a little flower.

– Hans Christian Andersen

The Princess was feeling misled by the White Witch by the time she started lesson two on the beginning of the end of her journey.

She had listened to the Broken Princesses tell their tales of Punishments and Captured Minds and Snakes and Shadows by their own Evil Kings. But as she listened, she realised that they were speaking about themselves as adults, not children.

The Princess shrank into herself and felt the creep of Shame across her Body. How could she tell her story about the Little Princess and the Evil King?

How shameful, they would think. *How dirty. How different. How very unnatural.*

And she shrank into herself at the very thought and kept quiet.

Afterwards, she spoke angrily to the White Witch.

'Why trick me?' she exclaimed. 'These people aren't like me at all! They look like me, they sound like me but I'm different! You can't help me!'

Once again, the Princess felt alone inside her bubble of Shame. She told the White Witch that she wanted to leave. But as she stepped through the yellow door, a strange thing happened. The inside of the blossom tree had enveloped the Princess in a cloak of warmth and comfort but when she put one foot out of the door, her Body was hit by an icy blast of air and freezing needles of sleet hurt her skin. the Princess felt unsettled. She turned and looked back at the White Witch. She saw that her face was kind, and her eyes were warm.

'Give it time,' she said gently, and the Princess found that she couldn't help but trust her and anyway, she didn't have a coat. She sat back down at the table.

The Transparent Princess took hold of the Princess's hand and the Princess could feel her poor, brittle bones through the skin. On her right, The Giantess reached for her other hand. One by one, the princesses joined hands. The Giantess held The Mute and the Mute held The Cut. The Cut held The Drowned and the White Witch, completing the circle, joined hands with the first princess and the last.

The White Witch looked warmly at the Princess and smiled a gentle smile of encouragement, and the Princess, taking a deep breath, closed her eyes and began to speak her story. She told of the Snakes and the Shadow. She told them about Mind Capture and Rules and Punishments. She told them about photographs and boxes and black doors with bolts and locks, and finally, she told them who the Evil King was.

The Princess waited and listened and there was silence inside the blossom tree, and she began to feel angry with the White Witch. She glanced at her and seeing her gentle smile, wanted to slap her and shake her until she turned back time and cast a spell to put the words back inside her mouth and she'd never speak of it again. But then, the Princess heard the most magical words.

'Me too,' said The Drowned.

And the words that had been spoken danced in the air and turned into tiny pink seeds that twirled and pirouetted in the air. Like dust motes, the little speckles of pink caught the light and the princesses watched as the White Witch held out her hands and let them settle gently on her palms. Then, she walked to the open yellow door, palms outstretched, stood, and waited. The wind died down and next came the birds. Flocks of colourful birds. Beautiful creatures of all colours glided and soared above, and one by one flew down, picked up a seed from the White Witch's palm in an elegant, curved beak, and flew back into the sky. the Princesses watched as the sky became full of colour. The ice and sleet had disappeared, the sun came out, and the beautiful birds with the little pink seeds dispersed in all directions.

'Where are they going?' asked the Princess.

The White Witch replied, 'There is a lot of work to be done. There are a lot of Broken Princesses in The World. Each bird will drop their seed and it will grow into a tree as beautiful as this one. And every tree will have a White Witch and the princesses will come from far and wide and find the trees, and when they too can speak the words then the birds will come again and pick up more seeds and plant more blossom trees.'

'But how can that help?' asked the Princess.

'Because,' the White Witch carried on, 'some of these seeds will land on different lands. There are many lands in The World and many Evil Kingdoms. Too many to count. The seeds will land, and the trees will grow, and the broken little Princesses will understand that they are not alone.'

The Princess was cynical. The Evil King would just have trodden on a beautiful seedling. He would have stamped it out before it even had a chance to begin.

'Yes,' said the White Witch patiently. 'He would, because that's what Monsters do. He would have squashed and killed it. But he wouldn't be able to, not entirely, because these seeds, these words are so powerful that once they've been released, they grow. They keep on growing, even when squashed and apparently dead. There's always a little root that continues to thrive, deep within the ground, and the seed will grow again, bigger, stronger, faster and more powerful, until one day there are so many words and so many seeds and so many blossom trees that the whole world will see them.

'The people in The World will ask, "What are these trees? Why are they so beautiful? Why are there so many? Why are they here?"

'And the Princesses will begin to speak. They will tell The World their terrible secrets. They will educate The World about Mind Capture. They will talk about Cold Ice Eyes and Rules. Punishments and Cats and Mice. Frozen Statues and Snakes. About Shadows of Rocks and delicious nectar. Because they will be together, they will be strong and they will talk about the lakes of wine and the swords and gardens of food.

'They will talk and talk and talk and at first, the people

won't want to hear their stories. "Not in my world," they will say, and some will put their fingers in their ears so as not to hear the terrible secrets.

'But one day, The World will be so full of these words, that the people will have to stop as they bump into them wherever they turn. They will trip over them and the people of The World will be forced to stop. And to listen.

'And the Evil Kings will begin to feel the first stirrings of fear; a feeling they have never felt before.

'They will pretend of course. "How terrible," they will lament. "What Evil people walk amongst us." But their voices will begin to catch and tremble. And The People will notice. They will begin to look. They will begin to watch and wonder, and the Evil Kings will find it harder and harder to do the things that they love to do.'

The Princess was silent.

She thought about the Butterfly Queen, who had been too busy to stop and notice the Evil King. She had heard the stories about other Little Princesses who lived on their islands with an Evil King and an Evil Queen too. She had heard about Little Princes and Evil Aunts and Evil Grandfathers and Evil Uncles and she wondered, *What about them? Who will care enough to watch and look and listen?*

And the White Witch heard the Little Princess's wondering and carried on.

'The Teachers,' she said. 'The Doctors, The Social Workers, the friends, the neighbours. They too have ears and must listen to this story. They have eyes to watch and see, and they will have the knowledge that they didn't have before.

'These are Very Powerful Words,' said the White Witch. 'You just need to learn how to speak them. It won't always be easy. Sometimes you may speak so many words that you will run out entirely and you will need to sit and be still and wait to feel strong again. At other times, it may hurt your heart to speak the words and you may feel like giving up. That is why there needs to be so many of you. The more of you there are, the stronger you become and the weaker and more frightened the Evil Kings will become, until, one day, they won't be able to hide their secrets anymore. There will be too many words and too many ears and too many eyes, watching, listening – not only to them, but to their own Little Prince and Princesses, for signs of these terrible crimes.'

The Princess felt tired. She felt that she couldn't do this important work. She was too tired and too broken. She needed time to sleep first.

'Yes,' said the White Witch. 'Give it time. First, it's time to heal.' And she lay the Princesses down on a comfortable bed of blossom, and she fed them fragrant blossom tea and nourishing blossom cake and the Princesses closed their weary eyes.

'I'm going to tell you a story,' said the White Witch.

And she told them a sad story about a Little Princess and an Evil King, and the Princesses cried because the story was so sad.

Then she told them about a Beautiful Queen and her Evil Husband, and they cried some more.

She talked about Evil Queens too and Little Princes, and they heard about the Shame and Fear and Humiliation and Revulsion. They listened to these stories and they cried and cried until they had no more tears left.

'You have trusted me so far, now you need to trust me a little bit more. I have noticed it is common for broken princesses to loathe themselves. It is usual for them to regret the way they reacted in the past. Sometimes, this loathing and regret is turned inwards. You harm yourselves, your bodies, and your minds. It is not you that you should be loathing and regretting.

'You want your mind and soul to be released. Every time you go to criticise and harm yourselves, I want you to imagine doing that to each other. You wouldn't. Next, you will need to accept what happened to you and find Words to put to the vile acts you had no words for as Little Princesses. You will find that they will stick in your throat, at first. They will choke you, because that is how powerful they are. These are important words and people in The World will need to hear them and hear your stories, to realise the horror of Evil Kings and to learn the importance of opening their Eyes and their Ears.'

So, the Princesses put their heads together and began to slowly whisper the horrible Words. The White Witch was right. They were Ugly Words, full of angles and points and they were painful to speak. They stuck in their throats and scraped against the tender skin of their mouths and made them vomit

and cry, but the Princesses were determined and brave and didn't give up. They spoke The Words over and over, louder and louder until they began to feel softer and malleable and could slip out of their mouths easily. These words were:
    Child Sexual Abuse
    Molestation
    Psychological abuse
    Narcissism
    Physical abuse
    Sadism
    Child abuse
    Coercive control
    Physical abuse
    Paedophile
    Psychopathy
    Sexual assault
    Grievous bodily harm
    Torture
    And Rape.

Some Princesses had experienced one of those Words, others many on the list. For some, it was a father who had inflicted the pain. For others, it was a partner/husband/mother/brother/teacher. the Princess understood that it didn't matter. The impact of this abuse was the same.

She saw that the Evil King had stolen the most precious parts of her. He had stolen her self-belief and self-worth, self-assurance, self-love and courage. He had taken away her innocence, her ability to trust, to see colour, to feel joy and to look forward. He had robbed her of a childhood but, in a beautiful paradox, the taking had given the Princess a power. She had the ability to look beneath the surface, to step back and observe, the ability to feel empathy, a finely tuned instinct and a strong sense of survival, even during times that she'd wanted to die. The Princess began to understand that she wasn't Stupid and Useless and Weak at all, and she never had been. She saw the Evil King's plans had been flawed all along.

Dark follows Light but she'd forgotten that Light follows Dark.

The Princess could feel this power now. She could feel it in her toes, it was bubbling in her legs and surging through her

Body. It ran through her veins and arteries and it filled her heart and head and soul.

She could see the White Witch looking into her soul with her wise, warm eyes and she knew that the White Witch was seeing it too. She nodded at the Princess and the Princess smiled.

She looked at the words, visible, and suspended above the heads of the women who had spoken them. They were Ugly, Grey words. The other Princesses looked fearfully at the words and at each other.

'No shame,' the White Witch reminded them.

'No shame,' they reminded each other and themselves.

'These words were done to you. You didn't have a choice. This happened to you.'

'It was not my fault,' whispered one Princess.

'I never asked for this,' said the next.

'I said no,' said another.

'Me too.'

'I tried to stop him.'

and

'I said nothing at all,' said the Princess, in a clear, loud voice, 'and it was not my fault. It is not my shame.'

And they watched as the hard, Ugly Words began to change colour and shape. They became softer and brighter and began to dance and shimmer in the air above until, *pop!* Each word turned into a little pink seed and the Princesses laughed and caught the seeds in their outstretched hands.

The Princesses walked to the open yellow door and stood and waited. Again, the flock of colourful birds came swooping down, each one picking up a seed from their outstretched palms.

The Princess felt lighter. She felt her Shadow of Rocks withering and dying. She stamped her feet and jumped up and down until the final piece fell away, then she trampled on the broken fragments with her princess feet, crunching and crushing, smashing and crumbling, until a pile of black dust was all that was left. She fetched a dustpan and a brush and she carefully swept, swept, swept, before tipping the dust into the bin.

The Princess knew that her journey had come to an end.

Her soul was free, and she finally understood her Purpose. She settled down in the blossom tree, with the White Witch and the Princesses, and they made themselves another pot of tea and waited for the new blossom trees to grow.

Not The End

Epilogue

Autumn 2023

The Flying Child is now an established Community Interest Company (CIC), and our professional training, The Flying Child Project, brings lived experience into the heart of professional and educational settings. Often I receive the inevitable question – how are you now? – and feel a moment of guilt that I can't allay the fears, that there is no fairy tale happy ending – or at least not the one they might be hoping for. 'Well . . .' I begin, 'life is a lot easier than it was, that's for sure, but you don't leave it behind. It's not that simple.'

If it *was* that simple then there would be no need for survivor activism, for accessible pathways or for trauma-informed practice. There would be no campaigning to have our needs recognised and not victim blamed, misunderstood or labelled as reflective of something inherently *wrong* with us.

The consequences of trauma are what they are, and there's no escaping that. I still get triggered at times, although significantly less than I did before. I still have flashbacks and suffer from nightmares. I am so traumatised by accessing medical care that when I have no choice, it can tip me into a state of abject fear. I can lose my voice entirely.

My husband who acts as my advocate does his best to help practitioners understand that no, this is not a mental health crisis – *No, it's not a psychiatrist she needs, it is a trauma responsive approach. She needs empathy, someone to understand her needs and offer a solution.* But he knows he is shouting into the wind – that all they see are the labels on my notes – *severe and enduring* – and it becomes a battle of wills and a battle he should not have to have. At times he does everything he can to prevent me from losing autonomy and has had to beg for compassionate care – hoping to find just one person who gets it (they are out there).

When I receive the care I need, I recover very quickly, often within hours, and it's frightening to think that without this advocacy, I am at risk of my distress being so misunderstood that I might even be sectioned – because of history of mental illness on my notes.

If this was to happen to me, I doubt whether I'd be OK after 28 days in a psychiatric ward. There is only so much trauma one can survive.

It frightens me that I live with these labels on my notes and one day I would like to challenge the diagnoses I was given, for it to be acknowledged that they were wrong – not that I've made some sort of miraculous and spontaneous recovery, but that *they were wrong* in the first place. I would like my labels removed. I believe in my case trauma was misunderstood as illness.

My physical health remains poor and probably always will. My condition is degenerative, and the grim prognosis includes terms such as *intractable pain, pressure on heart and lungs*, and *life limiting*, but maybe they're wrong. I was told at fifteen I'd be unable to have children because of my condition, but I have had four. All born naturally, at home, with no pain relief. Four little fuck yous to a system that doesn't recognise my needs. Maybe I'll be OK. Perhaps one day I will find the trauma responsive team I need to support me through major spinal surgery, but I suspect it's unlikely I will see the necessary changes within the medical system within my own lifetime. In the meantime I manage pain to the best of my ability, without medical help, because it is currently inaccessible to me as a survivor of Child Sexual Abuse.

I do believe CSA survivors can find a way to live alongside trauma, but it's not easy. When asked, I explain that I feel lucky, as a multiple suicide survivor, to be here at all – and that I view my eldest children as indirect victims of CSA too, because of bearing witness to this aftermath of trauma. No child should have to go through that. No child should have to witness a parent being tended to by paramedics. Children shouldn't have to visit their mother in a psychiatric ward. But one thing is for certain: because I was lucky to find Pat, the trauma now *ends with me*. We are doing well. There is joy to be found in life, sometimes it just takes us longer than feels fair to find it.

I hesitate to use the word 'recovery' because I think the word erases the seriousness of living with this specific type of sexual violence through the suggestion of an end point, which there's not. I will always be impacted by Child Sexual Abuse. If I have to use the word, then I redefine it. 'Recovery', for me, means that I no longer live with shame, suicidal ideation or rely on adverse coping mechanisms to get through the day.

It is being able to be myself and not hide what happened either from myself or others.

'Recovery' is being able to say, *I am a survivor,* without shame.

It is accepting that I might sometimes fall backwards for a while, but when triggered, 'recovery' is not reaching for a bottle of wine (or worse) to chase the body memories away. If I do, that doesn't mean I've failed. 'Recovery' means I will try again tomorrow.

'Recovery' is being able to voice my needs that are a direct result of trauma, without guilt or shame.

It is knowing for sure that 'normal' life is for me too, not just for other people.

I'm proud of where I am today and for the organisation I have created and I'll be forever grateful to the ones who played an important role – who advised me, mentored and supported me – who said, *keep going... your story is important... this is important.* I'm grateful because *all* of this – the book, the Flying Child Project, the non-profit, the activism – *is* my healing.

I needed to hear their words of encouragement and it's not exactly easy to express that need without sounding terribly insecure and, well... *needy*. It costs nothing to be kind and we won't know what positive impact it might have on a person. Kindness and encouraging words might take the sting out of the fear, be the healing balm for wounds, caused by the cut of not-so-kind words from a time past.

Because of trauma resulting from abuse, I had lost my sense of self and I didn't know what I was capable of. I believed in what I was doing but I didn't always believe in myself. I would doubt myself. *What right do I have to do any of this? Surely the right to educate others is earned through academic study? Is it not dictated by doctorates or degrees, by the letters after our names?* I didn't have these. I should have, I was capable, but trauma was a thief, and opportunity was snatched from my grasp. Surviving CSA and its legacy had taken priority.

Self-doubt is insidiously destructive and there were times over the last few years when I wondered if it would be easier to give up on my vision, but I recalled the kind words, the encouragement. *Keep going. This is important. It's valuable work.* I reassured myself I was offering people the chance to understand the nuanced complexities of CSA, silence and stigma, through the eyes of the survivor.

Today, I work with colleagues, researchers and academics, survivor activists, charities, professionals and practitioners across different sectors, and I see the power of working as one to move this forward. We all have a role to play in making The World a better place.

Sometimes in my life I'm struck by the fortuitous timings of events and how something seemingly inconsequential triggers a chain reaction. It is a feeling of – dare I say it – that some things are meant to be. Apart from CSA. That, of course, is *never* meant to be.

Had I not attended the safeguarding session and decided to speak to Clare afterwards . . . Had I not said the words *I was one of those children* . . . Had she not been professionally curious, we would not have had a conversation. I might not have realised the power of first-hand experience and The Flying Child Project, which led to the setup of the CIC, might not have existed at all.

Without Pat I wouldn't have found my lost words in the first place. They would not have been read and listened to by other survivors and professionals, including by one person who decided ours was the organisation they believed in and instigated a ball rolling that led to a large donation. We are National Lottery Community Funded, as they have recognised the value of our work, and are running peer support for adult CSA survivors across the world. Our groups are designed and co-led by survivors, partly because I believe it is important to set the example that not only is there life beyond CSA, it is possible to use our experiences to make a difference *and even get paid for it*. These groups bring much needed hope.

> 'I would describe the group as "a light at the end of a dark tunnel". The group is supportive and kind. Your feelings and thoughts are welcomed and supported. For me, the group gave me strength and purpose to carry on and to not give up. For me, seeing Sophie be in the place she is in today, knowing she was in similar position of wanting to give up back then, gave me hope. This group's made me realise that I can get out of this dark tunnel. It will be a journey, and not an easy one, but it is possible. Before this group I thought it wasn't achievable. So, I can recommend this group by saying I truly believe it has saved me and set me on a new path for the rest of my life.'
>
> The Flying Child peer group participant

Perhaps someone will read this book and fund the first Flying

Child specialist support centre for survivors of CSA, a place for survivors to step out of life for a while and have the chance to 'just be'. To remove the mask, to be held by a multitude of highly trained 'Pats'. Somewhere where flashbacks are allowed to happen, and traumatic memory is supported, not suppressed with benzodiazepines, antidepressants, and antipsychotics. This would be a place where it is not considered boundary crossing to be fully present with a client twenty-four hours a day, but recognised as a necessary part of the therapeutic process – a trauma intensive care. A place where coping mechanisms are recognised for what they really are – survival.

This centre would be a beautiful place with open space, healing views – where you could see the sky. Hear the birds. A place to bring colour back into the lives of people living in Grey, held back by the Shadow of Rocks. A place of acceptance, empathy and understanding. A place to put fragmented souls back together again, where you can learn how to laugh, to rage, to cry, to grieve for a childhood lost. A place to heal.

In your dreams, you might be thinking – especially if you're a practitioner in the overstretched and underfunded NHS, but let me reframe it for you. This open letter was composed by Patrick Sandford – a Survivor Activist and creator of the play, 'Groomed'. It was a letter I gladly put my name to.

Dear Editor,
The United Kingdom is facing a devastating financial crisis. Here is one potentially effective way forward to help reduce the debt.
The recent final report (20.10.22) of the Independent Inquiry into Childhood Sexual Abuse highlights that:
'In December 2021, the Home Office published a study into the costs relating to children whose contact sexual abuse began or continued in the year ending March 2019. The estimated cost to society exceeded £10 billion.' This figure is only for England and Wales. Our prisons, psychiatric hospitals, unemployment offices, social security offices are filled with adult survivors of Childhood Sexual Abuse. Make no mistake, Child Sexual Violation is a pandemic every bit as widespread as Covid 19, and it costs us more.
Today, November 18th, is approved by the United Nations as World Day for the Prevention of, and Healing from, Child Sexual Exploitation, Abuse and Violence. UK and World leaders at both National and Local Government Level would do well to start

addressing immediately this costly pandemic. Frankly, it's a no-brainer. 1 in 7 of our children currently experience sexual abuse before the age of 16. The damage can be lifelong – to productivity, social engagement, and happiness. Not investing to prevent this abuse, and to heal survivors, would be the equivalent of not researching a vaccine or treatment for Covid 19. To ignore this means of saving £ billions, would be grossly irresponsible.

Yours sincerely

So, yes, properly funded centres would cost millions, but so does the current, overwhelmed mental health system. So many people never leave it and, whilst this might suit some, it isn't right for all, and certainly doesn't suit the NHS. I wonder how many CSA survivors are, like I was, trapped in the endless cycle of crisis care? I wonder how much Pat has single-handedly saved the NHS through her support of me.

The number of professionals we have trained in a little over a year is now in the thousands. We have signposted many survivors for support.

Because of our work, there will be a greater likelihood of professionals who take time to ask, to consider trauma as the underlying cause of the behaviour, to not victim blame, shame or turn away from human distress. A greater chance of wondering *why* and not inadvertently shutting the child or adult down simply because they cannot hide their own fear or disgust. There will be a greater likelihood of the survivor being recognised, signposted, receiving specialist help, meeting other survivors and of realising they are, in fact, not alone – that their trauma responses are not something to feel ashamed of. As the activist Viv Gordon would say, *They should be celebrated as a creative act of survival.*

So, in answer to the question, *How are you now?* I'm doing well. I'm not an onlooker to my own life. I am living it. I hope my children see me as an emotionally present (albeit busy) mother. A role model. I look forward to seeing all my children grow, to having grandchildren one day. I couldn't look to the future before I met Pat and now I can. Trauma never goes away but it is possible to transform some of the pain into a light that guides others, and in doing so, empower ourselves. The Flying Child CIC is an organisation that helps others, but it continues to be my healing. It is my justice; it is my light.

Acknowledgements

I would like to say a huge thank you to all the survivors who have helped to shape and deliver The Flying Child Project, and the schools, institutions and individuals I have worked with. I hope this book is instrumental in extending my work across the UK and beyond.

With special thanks to my friends and family who have supported me along the way, my husband who is the most supportive and kindest one in the world, my beautiful three sons and one daughter, and also the following:

Elaine Bousfield for being the best editor and working with kindness and compassion, and her colleagues at ZunTold Publishing who all played an important part in the design and production.

Jemima Foxtrot for lending me her agent and to Charlotte Colwill for the fairest deal in literary history.

Leah Price-Cox, Dr Clare Brunet, Dr Charlotte Small, Jo Watson, Sarah Pritchard and Redzi Bernard, for having faith and opening doors.

Alex O'Donnell for his advice: 'Just take them on a journey.'

Catherine Cox, Rhianna Fairfax, Vicki Balaam, Kate Alger, Claire Bloor and John Slater for generous help and advice.

Saša Janković for giving me the confidence to start blogging, Clare Shaw and Sur5vor for showing me poetry is the opposite of boring and giving me tools to make sense of my experience on days where survival is more challenging.

The CSA activists who inspire me along the way, with thanks to Viv Gordon for being the first person who made me reflect on (and value) my worth in this space.

Academics and researchers for respectfully inviting me into their space or graciously accepting the invite into mine.

The National Lottery Community Fund and to the person who decided ours was the organisation they would like to donate to – your decision is changing lives. Thank you.

And to Pat, just – thank you. I have no need to complete 'The Suit of Clothes' exercise, for they were the clothes I was wearing all along. Because of you, I am free to be me.

For other insightful books,

head to

Zuntold.com

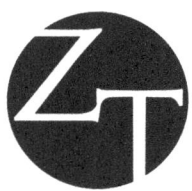